MRCP PART 1 PRACTICE EXAMS

Edited by

P. ACKRILL MB. ChB. FRCP.

MRCP PART 1
PRACTICE EXAMS

Edited by
P. ACKRILL MB. ChB. FRCP.

© 1985 PASTEST SERVICE.
Cranford Lodge, Bexton Road, Knutsford, Cheshire WA16 0ED.
Telephone: 0565 55226

First published 1982 large format
Reprinted 1985
Reprinted 1986
Reprinted and updated 1989

British Library Cataloguing in Publication Data

Ackrill, P.
MRCP part 1 : practice exams.
  1. Medicine – Problems, exercises, etc.
  610'.76   R834.5

  ISBN 0-906896-16-9

Text prepared using an Apple Microcomputer.
Phototypeset by Designed Publications using an interface.
Printed by Martins of Berwick.

CONTENTS

FOREWORD   v

EXAMINATION TECHNIQUE   vi

MULTIPLE CHOICE QUESTION PAPERS

INSTRUCTIONS   x

     Practice Exam 1   1
     Practice Exam 2   16
     Practice Exam 3   31
     Practice Exam 4   46
     Practice Exam 5   62

ANSWERS AND TEACHING EXPLANATIONS

     Practice Exam 1   77
     Practice Exam 2   88
     Practice Exam 3   99
     Practice Exam 4   110
     Practice Exam 5   121

RECOMMENDED READING AND REFERENCE LIST   134

MCQs LISTED BY SUBJECT   137

MCQ REVISION INDEX   139

SAMPLE COMPUTER ANSWER CARD   145

FOREWORD

The MRCP examination has been an unavoidable hurdle for generations of aspiring physicians in this country and overseas. The introduction of multiple choice questions in Part I of the exmination has enabled those hostile agencies, the examiners, to probe more deeply and widely than before into the candidates' data-bank of knowledge and the candidate must therefore arm himself appropriately for this encounter. Although each must individually develop the pattern of work most suited to his temperament and opportunities for study, most will find the Pastest system invaluable in sharpening their critical attitudes to the torments of the MCQ. It should be particularly useful in revealing areas of deficient knowledge which can then be remedied by recourse to the appropriate texts.

Yet the candidates must never forget that the examination overall is a test of clinical competence in the whole field of general medicine.

Although wide reading of text books and journals is obviously an essential part of this preparation, the candidate's fate will be decided by whether or not he is able to convince experienced clinicians that he can take an excellent history from the patient, can competently examine the various systems, and can make reasonable deductions from a body of clinical and non-clinical data. To this end, even while preparing for Part I of the examination, it is essential that the candidate develops his clinical expertise. The best way to do this is to obtain a busy senior house officer or registrar post in a clinical unit that is not too specialised, and which gives the doctor the opportunity of seeing a wide range of medical in-patients and out-patients. The actual exercise of clinical responsibility (always provided that the doctor has someone more experienced to consult when he feels out of his depth) is the best way to acquire that level of competence which befits a Member of the Royal College of Physicians.

Attendance at postgraduate courses, although often excellent in themselves, is no substitute for hard-won clinical experience. It is a mistake to separate too rigidly the service and training aspects of junior medical posts; the young doctor learns as he acutally does the work – a system of clinical apprenticeship which has served this country's doctors well for generations.

It goes without saying that time for study and revision in such a post will not be great; this should be a matter of satisfaction rather than regret but it does of course mean that the little time available must be used to the best effect. It is in the belief that the present volume will amply serve such a purpose that it is warmly commended.

J. C. LEONARD, MD FRCP
Consultant Physician
Withington Hospital
Manchester

Multiple Choice Questions are the most reliable, reproducible and internally consistent method we have of testing re-call of factual knowledge. Yet there is evidence that they are able to test more than simple factual re-call; reasoning ability and an understanding of basic facts, principles and concepts can also be assessed. A good MCQ paper will discriminate accurately between candidates on the basis of their knowledge of the topics being tested. It must be emphasised that the most important function of an MCQ paper of the type used in the MRCP Part 1, is to rank candidates accurately and fairly according to their performance in that paper. Accurate ranking is the key phrase; this means that all MCQ examinations of this type are, in a sense, competitive.

Technique

The safest way to pass Part 1 MRCP is to know the answers to all of the questions, but it is equally important to be able to transfer this knowledge accurately onto the answer sheet. All too often, candidates suffer through an inability to organise their time, through failure to read the instructions carefully or through failure to read and understand the questions. First of all you must allocate your time with care. There are 60 questions to complete in 2½ hours; this means 2½ minutes per question or 10 questions in 25 minutes. Make sure that you are getting through the exam at least at this pace, or, if possible, a little quicker, thus allowing time at the end for revision and a re-think on some of the items that you have deferred.

You must read the question (both stem and items) carefully. You should be quite clear that you know what you are being asked to do. Once you know this, you should indicate your responses by marking the paper boldly, correctly and clearly. Take great care not to mark the wrong boxes and think very carefully before making a mark on the answer sheet.

Regard each item as being independent of every other item, each refers to a specific quantum of knowledge. The item (or the stem and the item taken together) make up a statement. You are required to indicate whether you regard this statement as 'True' or 'False' and you are also able to indicate 'Don't know'. Look only at a single statement when answering, disregard all the other statements presented in the question. They have nothing to do with the item you are concentrating on.

Marking your answer sheets

The answer sheet will be read by an automatic document reader, which transfers the information it reads to a computer. It must therefore be filled out in accordance with the instructions. A sample of the answer sheet, together with the instructions, is printed in the booklet of Examination Regulations available from the Royal Colleges. Study these instructions carefully, well before the exams, the invigilators will also draw attention to them at the time of the examination. You must first fill in your name on the answer sheet, and then fill in your examination number. It is critical that this is filled in correctly. At present, page numbers must also be filled in, but in the future, it is possible that newly-designed sheets may remove the need for this step.

As you go through the questions, you can either mark your answers immediately on the answer sheet, or you can mark them in the question book first of all, transferring them to the answer sheets at the end. If you adopt the second approach, you must take great care not to run out of time, since you will not be allowed extra time to transfer marks to the answer sheet from the question book. The answer sheet must always be marked neatly and carefully according to the instructions given. Careless marking is probably one of the commonest causes of rejection of answer sheets by the document reader. For although the computer operator will do his best to interpret correctly the answer you intended, and will then correct the sheet accordingly, the procedure introduces a possible new source of error. You are, of course, at liberty to change your mind by erasing your original selection and selecting a new one. In this event, your erasure should be carefully, neatly, and completely carried out.

Try to leave time to go over your answers again before the end, in particular going back over any difficult questions that you wish to think about in more detail. At the same time, you can check that you have marked the answer sheet correctly. However, repeated review of your answers may in the end be counter-productive, since answers that you were originally confident were absolutely correct, often look rather less convincing at a second, third or fourth perusal. In this situation, first thoughts are usually best and too critical a revision might lead you into a state of confusion.

To guess or not to guess

Do not mark at random. Candidates are frequently uncertain whether or not to guess the answer. However, a clear distinction must be made between a genuine guess (i.e. tails for True, heads for False) and a process of reasoning by which you attempt to work out an answer that is not immediately apparent by using first principles and drawing on your knowledge and experience. Genuine guesses should not be made. You might be lucky, but if you are totally ignorant of the answer, there is an equal chance that you will be wrong and thus lose marks. This is not a chance that is worth taking, and you should not hesitate to indicate 'Don't know' if this genuinely and honestly expresses your view.

Although you should not guess, you should not give in too easily. What you are doing is to increase as much as possible the odds that the answer you are going to give is the correct one, even though you are not

100% certain that this is the case. Take time to think, therefore, drawing on first principles and reasoning power, and delving into your memory stores. Do not, however, spend an inordinate amount of time on a single item that is puzzling you. Leave it, and, if you have time, return to it. If you are 'fairly certain' that you know the right answer or have been able to work it out, it is reasonable to mark the answer sheet accordingly. There is a difference between being 'fairly certain' (odds better than 50:50 that you are right) and totally ignorant (where any response would be a guess). The phrase 'MCQ technique' is often mentioned, and is usually used to refer specifically to this question of 'guessing' and 'Don't know'. Careful thought and reasoning ability, as well as honesty, are all involved in so-called 'technique', but the best way to increase the odds that you know the right answers to the questions, is to have a sound basic knowledge of medicine and its specialties.

Trust the examiners
Do try to trust the Examiners. Accept each question at its face value, and do not look for hidden meanings, catches and ambiguities. Multiple Choice Questions are not designed to trick or confuse you, they are designed to test your knowledge of medicine. Don't look for problems that aren't there - the obvious meaning of a statement is the correct one and the one that you should read.

Candidates often try to calculate their score as they go through the paper; their theory is that if they reach a certain score they should then be safe in indicating 'Don't know' for any items that they have left blank without needing to take the trouble to think out answers. This approach is not to be recommended. No candidate can be certain what score he will need to achieve to obtain a pass in the examination, and everyone will overestimate the score he thinks he has obtained by answering questions confidently. The best approach is to answer every question honestly and to make every possible effort to work out the answers to more difficult questions, leaving the 'Don't know' option to indicate exactly what it means. In other words, your aim should always be to obtain the highest possible score on the MCQ paper.

To repeat the four most important points of technique:

(1) Read the question carefully and be sure you understand it.
(2) Mark your responses clearly, correctly and accurately.
(3) Use reasoning to work out answers, but if you do not know the answer and cannot work it out, indicate 'Don't know'.
(4) The best way to obtain a good mark is to have as wide a knowledge as possible of the topics being tested in the examination.

John Anderson MB. BS. FRCP.
The Medical School
Newcastle-upon-Tyne.

ACKNOWLEDGEMENTS

A sincere thankyou is due to the many doctors in the Greater Manchester area whose advice & contributions have made this book possible:

Peter Barnes, Steve Shalet, Ken Cummings, Ian Burton, Peter Whorwell, Gary Hambledon, John Mackay, George Mawer, Edward Dunbar and Gregory Summers.

INSTRUCTIONS

In order to help MRCP Part I candidates revise for this difficult examination we have tried to follow as closely as possible the content and format of the official examination. Each question has an answer and teaching explanation which should provide a good basis for successful revision.

We suggest that you work on each set of 60 multiple choice questions as though it was a real examination. In other words time yourself to spend no more than 2½ hours on each practice exam and do not obtain help from books, notes or persons while working on each test. Plan to take this practice exam at a time when you will be undisturbed for a minimum of 2½ hours. Choose a well lit location free from distractions, keep your desk clear of other books or papers, have a clock or watch clearly visible with a rubber and 2 well sharpened grade B pencils to hand.

As you work through each question in this book be sure and mark a tick or cross (True or False) against the A... B... C... D... E... answer space below each question. If you do not know the answer then leave the answer space blank. Thus when you have completed the paper you can mark your own answers with the help of the answers and explanations given at the end of the book. Do not be tempted to look at the questions before sitting down to take each test as this will not then represent a mock exam.

When you have finished an exam be sure to go back over your answers until the 2½ hours is over. When your time is up you can then mark your answers and study the teaching explanations carefully so as to learn from your mistakes. Give yourself+ 1 for every correct answer,–1 for every incorrect answer and 0 for an unanswered (don't know) question. Put a mark clearly the book wherever you put a wrong answer and this will help you with your final revision as the official exam grows near.

Good luck with your revision.

PRACTICE EXAM 1

60 Questions: time allowed 2½ hours.

1 The following statements are true of primary pulmonary tuberculosis:

A with symptomless primary complex, gastric washings are required to isolate myobacteria
B spontaneous healing is the typical outcome
C chemotherapy is normally recommended
D miliary tuberculosis may occur
E it is usually symptomless

Your answers: A.......B........C.......D.......E........

2 Exophthalmos due to Graves' disease

A may be present when the patient is euthyroid
B may be unilateral
C may cause exposure keratitis
D always responds to high dose corticosteroids
E frequently improves spontaneously

Your answers: A.......B.......C.......D.......E........

3 The following are features of acute nephritis in the elderly:

A polyuria
B symptoms and signs of congestive cardiac failure
C elevated serum complement
D diarrhoea and vomiting
E hypokalaemia

Your answers: A.......B.......C.......D.......E........

4 Recognised features of Paget's disease of bone include

A hypercalcaemia
B nerve deafness
C angioid streaks in the retina
D brainstem compression
E osteoporosis

Your answers: A... ...B... ...C... ...D.......E........

5 **The following are recognised features of Wilson's disease:**

A   retinitis pigmentosa
B   low urinary copper
C   liver disease resembling chronic active hepatitis
D   reduced plasma caeruloplasmin
E   osteomalacia

Your answers: A.. ..B.. ...C.. ...D.....E.......

6 **The aortic arch**

A   is developed from the third left pharyngeal arch artery
B   is crossed anteriorly on the left by the vagus and phrenic nerves
C   is in communication with the pulmonary vein in the fetus
D   lies in both the superior and posterior mediastinum
E   arches backwards over the left main bronchus

Your answers: A.......B. ...C.......D.......E.. ...

7 **Which of the following statements are true of chemotherapy in tuberculosis:**

A   rifampicin turns the urine red 4-8 hours after ingestion
B   the incidence of hepatotoxicity has made isoniazid unacceptable as a first line drug
C   PAS can be detected in the urine by 'phenistix' paper strips
D   ethambutol blood levels are not significantly affected by renal insufficiency
E   isoniazid may lead to failure of the contraceptive pill

Your answers: A.. ..B.......C.. ...D.......E.......

8 **The following statements are true of Duchenne muscular dystrophy:**

A   it is inherited as an autosomal dominant
B   the serum creatinine phosphokinase levels are normal
C   an early manifestation may be frequent falls
D   muscular pseudohypertrophy is a feature
E   myotonia is characteristic

Your answers: A.......B.......C.... .D... ..E.......

9 **Thrombosis of the posterior inferior cerebellar artery causes**

A   speech impairment (dysphasia)
B   loss of pain and temperature sensation on the same side of the face
C   loss of pain and temperature sensation on the opposite side of the body
D   palatal palsy
E   double vision (diplopia)

Your answers: A.. ...B... ..C.. ..D...…..E.......

10 **The following are characteristic of anorexia nervosa:**

A   amenorrhoea
B   occurrence in pre-puberty girls
C   it never occurs in males
D   loss of body hair
E   purpura

Your answers: A.. ...B.......C......D.......E......

11 **The following diseases are associated with an increased liability to fracture in the elderly:**

A   osteoporosis
B   osteomalacia
C   osteopetrosis
D   hyperostosis frontalis interna
E   osteitis deformans   (Pagets)

Your answers: A.. ..B... ..C.......D.......E.......

12 **The following are recognized features of hypothyroidism:**

A   menorrhagia
B   ascites
C   cerebellar ataxia
D   clubbing
E   normochromic anaemia

Your answers: A.......B.. ..C.. ...D.......E.. ...

(13) **Recognised features of Reiter's syndrome include**

A   balanitis xerotica obliterans
B   calcaneal spurs
C   posterior uveitis
D   sacro-iliitis
E   subungual keratosis

Your answers: A.......B.......C.......D... ..E.. ..

(14) **Which of the following are true of child battering:**

A   parents who batter their children are suffering from a psychotic illness
B   parents who batter their children often come from unhappy homes
C   most abused children show delayed speech development
D   affected children are usually otherwise well cared for
E   most cases occur in infancy and early childhood

Your answers: A.......B.. ..C.. .D.......E. ....

(15) **The following are recognised clinical manifestations of myasthenia gravis:**

A   wasting of proximal muscles
B   dysphagia
C   peripheral sensory loss
D   double vision
E   fluctuating symptoms

Your answers: A.......B.. ..C.......D. ...E. ...

(16) **Recognised findings in a Pancoast tumour are**

A   erosion of the first rib
B   ipsilateral Horner's syndrome
C   paralysis of muscles in the arm
D   pain in the arm radiating to the 4th and 5th fingers
E   gangrene of the fingers on the same side

Your answers: A.. ...B. ...C.. ...D. ....E.......

17 **Cholestatic jaundice occurs with**

A combined contraceptive steroids
B erythromycin estolate
C methyldopa
D prochlorperazine
E tetracycline

Your answers: A.... ..B.......C.......D.'....E.......

18 **The following are recognised findings in acromegaly:**

A hypercalcaemia
B low serum inorganic phosphate
C cardiomegaly
D sexual impotence
E galactorrhoea

Your answers: A.......B.......C.......D.. ....E.......

19 **In the carcinoid syndrome**

A episodic hypertension is a feature
B patients with bronchial tumours have the most severe flushing
C patients with bronchial tumours have left sided heart lesions
D survival is not usually more than 10 years
E pellagra-like skin lesions may occur

Your answers: A..... .B.. ..C.. ..D.......L... :..

20 **In leptospirosis**

A the onset is characteristically abrupt
B myalgia is a frequent early symptom
C splenomegaly is found in a majority of cases
D hepatic failure is a recognised complication
E the diagnosis may be made by blood culture

Your answers: A..'...B..<.... C.......D.......E...<...

21 **In syphilis**

A   the causative organism is *Treponema pertenue*
B   the incubation period is typically 17-28 days
C   the ulcer of the primary stage is usually tender
D   a maculo papular rash is characteristic of the primary stage
E   serological tests are positive in the secondary stage

Your answers: A.......B.......C.......D.......E.......

22 **A radial nerve lesion above the elbow leads to**

A   paralysis of the extensor muscles of the wrist
B   inability to supinate the forearm
C   paralysis of the dorsal interossei
D   paralysis of the extensor pollicis brevis
E   sensory loss confined to the forearm

Your answers: A.......B.......C.......D.......E.......

23 **A low serum folate is a common finding in**

A   tropical sprue
B   pernicious anaemia
C   megaloblastic pregnancy anaemia
D   myxoedema
E   cirrhosis of the liver

Your answers: A.......B.......C.......D.......E.......

24 **Hyoscine is useful in preventing the nausea and vomiting associated with**

A   Meniere's disease
B   radiotherapy
C   motion sickness
D   pregnancy
E   cytotoxic agents

Your answers: A.......B.......C.......D.......L.......

25 Papilloedema

A   commonly produces concentric visual field loss
B   is a feature of benign intracranial hypertension
C   may occur in chronic bronchitis
D   occurs in malignant exophthalmic ophthalmoplegia
E   may be distinguished from pseudopapilloedema by fluoroscein angiography

Your answers: A... ..B.. ..C..:....D..'.....E.......

26 Insulin

A   is composed of an A and B chain
B   is broken down to C peptide
C   and C peptide are produced from Proinsulin
D   can cause a hypoglycaemia which may suppress growth hormone secretion.
E   release is inhibited by sulphonylureas

Your answers: A...: .B.......C..: ..D.......E.......

27 Which of the following findings are more suggestive of chronic ulcerative colitis than of granulomatous colitis (Crohn's disease):

A   'skip lesions' involving the small bowel
B   toxic dilatation of the colon
C   non-caseating granulomata in rectal biopsy
D   crypt abscesses on mucosal biopsy
E   fistulae

Your answers: A.......B..: ...C.......D...`..E.......

28 As compared with chronic myelocytic leukaemia, chronic lymphocytic leukaemia has

A   more marked lymphadenopathy
B   more frequent hypogammaglobulinaemia
C   a more frequent occurrence of a positive Coomb's test
D   more frequent development of a blast crisis
E   a worse prognosis

Your answers: A.. ..B.: ..C.. ...D.......E.......

29 **The following are recognised features of hyper-betalipoproteinaemia (hyper-cholesterolaemia):**

A   xanthomas
B   aortic stenosis
C   acute pancreatitis
D   corneal arcus
E   opalescent serum

Your answers: A...T..B...T...C.......D...T..E.......

30 **The following are true of chlamydial infections:**

A   they are caused by bacterial organisms
B   the organisms are sensitive to sulphonamides
C   they are a common cause of non-gonococcal urethritis in men
D   animals and birds are the primary hosts for some species
E   they are responsible for trichomoniasis

Your answers: A..T...B.......C..T...D..T..E.......

31 **The following structures are concerned with the light reflex:**

A   occipital cortex
B   optic nerve
C   lateral geniculate bodies
D   superior colliculi
E   third cranial nerve

Your answers: A.......B...T..C.......D.......E..T....

32 **In left ventricular failure therre is/are**

A   increased alveolar PCO_2
B   a decreased CO diffusion capacity
C   raised pulmonary venous pressure
D   reduced left ventricular end-diastolic pressure
E   basal crepitations heard before chest X-ray changes

Your answers: A.......B...T...C..T...D.......E.......

33 **Pulmonary abscess formation secondary to aspiration is characteristically seen in**

    A   basal segments of the lower lobes
    B   apical segments of the lower lobes
    C   anterior segments of the upper lobes
    D   posterior segments of the upper lobes
    E   the right lung more often than the left

Your answers: A.......B.......*C.......D....*....*E...*....

34 **Patients with idiopathic acquired autoimmune haemolytic anaemia**

    A   may have haemosiderinuria
    B   often have complicating folic acid deficiency
    C   show no recovery without specific therapy
    D   with rare exceptions, show complete response to splenectomy
    E   usually have an increase of both mechanical and osmotic fragility of red cells

Your answers: A.......B.......*C.......D...*...E...*....

35 **In severe acute poisoning**

    A   adequate pulmonary ventilation is the overriding priority
    B   coma need not be present for salicylate intoxication to threaten life
    C   forced diuresis shortens benzodiazepine induced coma
    D   naloxone fails to counteract pentazocine induced respiratory depression
    E   phenytoin is of value in digoxin intoxication

Your answers: A...T.B...T...C.......D.......E...T..

36 **In clinical trials which of the following are correct?**

    A   If the difference between treatments is not statistically significant "P greater than 0.05" then there is no clinically important difference between the treatments.
    B   Using the date of birth to randomise patients is not acceptable.
    C   In a single-blind trial the patient does not know the assigned treatment.
    D   If the sample size for each arm of a clinical trial is greater than 100 then randomisation is unnecessary.
    E   Randomising the allocation of treatments in a clinical trial guarantees that the characteristics of the patients in the different arms of the trial will be similar.

Your answers: A.......B...T...C.......D.......E.......

37 The following findings would suggest a diagnosis of coeliac disease:

A   a positive family history
B   Howell-Jolly bodies on the blood film
C   a normal serum folate
D   iron deficiency anaemia
E   a positive C14 breath test result

Your answers: A...T...B...T...C.......D..T...E.......

38 Pentazocine differs from codeine in that it

A   has higher analgesic efficacy
B   is less likely to induce dependence
C   is more likely to produce dysphoria
D   may occasionally cause visual hallucinations
E   should not be prescribed if there is any suspicion of opiate dependence

Your answers: A..T...B..T...C..T...D..T...E..T...

39 The following are features of Fallot's tetralogy:

A   squatting
B   syncopal attacks
C   systolic bruit due to ventricular septal defect
D   pulmonary oligaemia
E   cyanosis aggravated by exertion

Your answers: A..T...B..T...C.......D..T...E.T....

40 Seborrhoeic warts

A   are always multiple
B   are pre-malignant in many cases
C   are infective
D   never occur on the palms or soles
E   have a recognised association with internal malignancy

Your answers: A.......B.......C.......D..T...E.T....

41 **In Turner's syndrome, in a female aged 18**

A a buccal smear shows one Barr body
B she will be taller than average
C poor breast development is characteristic
D high urinary gonadotrophins are found
E uterine bleeding follows cyclic oestrogen-progestogen therapy

Your answers: A.......B.......C.∕...D..∕...E.∕...

42 **The following are features of encephalitis:**

A herpes simplex has a reasonably good prognosis in the young patient
B chickenpox encephalitis is predominantly 'cerebellar'
C herpes simplex predominantly affects the temporal lobe
D mumps encephalitis can cause unilateral nerve deafness
E herpes simplex can present as grand mal epilepsy

Your answers: A.......B..∕..C..∕..D..∕....E.∕....

43 **The classical rash of typhoid fever (rose spots)**

A occurs mainly on the face
B occurs during the first 2 weeks of illness
C usually lasts a week or more
D is petechial
E is commoner in paratyphoid than typhoid

Your answers: A.......B..T..C.......D.......E...T...

44 **Causes of nappy rash include**

A eczema
B candidiasis
C impetigo
D ammoniacal dermatitis
E herpes simplex

Your answers: A...T..B....T..C..T..D...T.E..T.......

45 **Urobilinogen in urine is**

A   not detectable in health
B   is only distinguishable from porphobilinogen by Ehrlich aldeyde reagent
C   diagnostic of intrahepatic obstruction
D   found to occur in pernicious anaemia
E   an indication of increased haemolysis

Your answers: A.......B.......C.......D...T...E..T....

46 **In chondrocalcinosis and pseudo-gout**

A   there is a significant association with hypothyroidism
B   the joint crystals are positively birefringent
C   intervertebral disc joints may be involved
D   males are more frequently affected
E   there is a significant association with haemochromatosis

Your answers: A.......B..T...C...T..D.......E..T....

47 **A 59 year old female presents with a serum calcium of 3.3 mmol/1., serum albumen 48 g/1., and a blood pressure of 190/100. The following statements are true:**

A   serum calcium is not raised because the serum albumen is high due to dehydration
B   a high serum parathormone would indicate a diagnosis of sarcoidosis
C   the initial treatment should be a thiazide diuretic
D   a low urinary calcium will indicate the presence of myeloma
E   diminished tubular re-absorption of phosphate would indicate the presence of a parathyroid adenoma

Your answers: A.......B.......C.......D.......E..T....

48 **Lung compliance is**

A   decreased by pulmonary congestion
B   a measure of change in lung volume per unit change in airway pressure
C   is decreased by emphysema
D   is approximately half in a person with only one lung
E   is determined using a peak flow meter

Your answers: A...T..B...T..C.......D...T..E.......

49 Conditions occurring as a result of chronic pancreatitis are

A steatorrhoea
B anorexia and weight loss
C diabetes mellitus
D pseudocyst formation
E osteomalacia

Your answers: A...T...B.......C....T..D..T..E..T...

50 Characteristic associations of temporal lobe epilepsy include

A deja vu experiences
B episodes of automatic behaviour
C feeling of detachment from surroundings
D 3 per second spike and wave pattern on the EEG
E perinatal trauma or anoxia

Your answers: A...T..B...F..C...F..D.......E..T...

51 In chronic constrictive pericarditis

A the patient is breathless at rest
B the jugular venous pulse rises on inspiration
C the jugular venous pulse falls markedly in early diastole
D calcification of the pericardium indicates a tuberculous aetiology
E peripheral oedema is prominent

Your answers: A.......B..T..C..T..D.......E.......

52 Calcified extra cardiac lesions on chest X-ray have a recognized association with

A asbestosis
B farmer's lung
C mitral stenosis
D silicosis
E chickenpox

Your answers: A..T..B.......C..T..D...T..E..T...

53   A falling haemoglobin with a 20% reticulocyte count may be due to

A   menorrhagia
B   congenital spherocytosis
C   sideroblastic anaemia
D   lead
E   methyldopa

Your answers: A.......B...T...C.......D...T...E...T...

54   Benzodiazepine anxiolytics differ significantly in their

A   anticonvulsant relative to anxiolytic activity
B   cost
C   duration of action
D   sedative relative to anxiolytic activity
E   muscle relaxant relative to anxiolytic activity

Your answers: A.......B...T...C...T...D.......E.......

55   In polymyalgia rheumatica

A   movement is restricted by pain rather than by muscular weakness
B   symptoms are characteristically worse at the end of the day
C   the muscles of the shoulder girdle are usually the first to be affected
D   the serum creatinine phosphokinase level is characteristically very greatly raised
E   the electromyogram is usually normal

Your answers: A...T...B.......C...T...D.......E...T...

56   Hypochondriasis can be an integral feature of the following illnesses:

A   schizophrenia
B   obsessive-compulsive neurosis
C   depression
D   dementia
E   anxiety state

Your answers: A...T..B..T...C...T..D...T..E.......

57 **The following statements are true of Infant Respiratory Distress Syndrome of prematurity:**

A   it does not occur after 36 weeks gestation
B   metabolic acidosis is the first physiological disturbance ·
C   it is associated with maternal diabetes mellitus
D   it is associated with sub-dural haemorrhage
E   it responds to corticosteroid therapy

Your answers: A.......B...1..C...1..D.......E.......

58 **In congestive cardiomyopathy the following features may be found:**

A   protodiastolic gallop   (3rd heart sound) ·
B   clinical improvement following intramuscular thiamine
C   mural thrombus formation
D   frequent arrhythmias, best treated with propranolol
E   pericardial effusion

Your answers: A..1...B..1..C...1..D.......E.......

59 **Bilateral basal crackles (crepitations) in the lungs are a typical finding in the following:**

A   emphysema due to alpha-1 antitrypsin deficiency
B   bronchiectasis following childhood whooping cough
C   pulmonary sarcoidosis
D   massive myocardial infarction
E   acute attack of bronchial asthma

Your answers: A.......B..1..C...1..D..1..E.......

60 **In patients with rheumatic fever the following indicate carditis:**

A   pericarditis
B   diastolic murmur
C   prolonged PR interval
D   sinus arrhythmia
E   cardiomegaly

Your answers: A..1..B..1..C.......D.......E..1..

| 08

END OF EXAM 1

Go over your answers until your time is up. Answers and explanations are on page 77.

Time allowed: 2½ hours ✓✓

1 The following statements are true concerning travellers' diarrhoea:

A an infective cause is rarely implicated
B the commonest pathogen is a toxin-producing strain of *E. coli*
C clioquinol (Enterovioform) causes a subacute myelo-optic neuropathy
D doxycycline is of prophylatic value
E predisposes to ulcerative colitis

Your answers: A.......B...F...C...T..D..T..E.......

2 A patient with longstanding bronchiectasis develops oedema; the following would support a diagnosis of amyloidosis:

A palpable spleen
B right ventricular hypertrophy
C clubbing of the fingers
D raised blood urea
E normal serum albumin

Your answers: A...T..B.......C.......D.......E.......

3 The headache of raised intracranial pressure

A tends to occur in the later part of the day
B is usually described as vice-like or gripping
C is made worse by coughing
D may be relieved by vomiting
E may be accompanied by episodes of transient blindness in both eyes

Your answers: A.......B...T..C..T..D...T..E...T...

4 Cannon waves in the jugular venous pulse are

A a special form of v-wave
B seen in complete heart block
C seen in tricuspid stenosis
D compatible with nodal rhythm
E associated with second degree heart block

Your answers: A.......B.......C.......D.......E.......

5 **Hyperuricaemia occurs in**

A   Lesch-Nyhan syndrome
B   polycythaemia rubra vera
C   primary hyperparathyroidism
D   starvation
E   thyrotoxicosis

Your answers: A.......B.......C.......D.......E.......

6 **Bromocriptine causes**

A   nausea and vomiting if taken on an empty stomach
B   a rise in serum growth hormone concentration in normal subjects
C   a fall in serum prolactin concentration
D   clinical improvement in some patients with acromegaly
E   a rise in plasma ACTH concentration in Cushing's syndrome

Your answers: A.......B.......C.......D.......E.......

7 **During normal heart action**

A   mitral valve closure occurs before tricuspid
B   a fourth heart sound is commonly audible during atrial systole
C   left atrial pressure has a waveform similar to jugular venous pressure
D   aortic valve cusps are immobile during ventricular filling
E   left ventricular stroke work is linearly related to left ventricular end-diastolic pressure

Your answers: A.......B.......C.......D.......E.......

8 **The following statement(s) is/are true of urinary infection in adults:**

A   *Proteus mirabilis* is the commonest offending organism in general practice
B   renal damage by analgesics is a predisposing factor
C   bladder neck obstruction predisposes to infection
D   bacterial colonisation of bladder urine is usually due to descending infection from the kidney
E   chronic renal failure is a common feature

Your answers: A.......B.......C.......D.......E.......

9 **The following are recognised complications of ulcerative colitis:**

A   acute colonic dilatation
B   amyloidosis
C   colonic perforation
D   arthritis
E   erythema nodosum

Your answers: A.......B.......C.......D.......E.......

10 **Coeliac disease**

A   is a life-long condition
B   is significantly associated with lactase deficiency
C   may present as iron deficiency anaemia
D   may present as acute diarrhoea and vomiting
E   requires jejunal biopsy for diagnosis

Your answers: A.......B.......C.......D.......E.......

11 **In dystrophia myotonica (myotonic dystrophy)**

A   the inheritance is X-linked
B   males only are affected
C   muscular weakness is initially marked in the distal muscles of the limbs
D   cardiac abnormalities occur
E   testicular atrophy occurs

Your answers: A.......B.......C.......D.......E.......

12 **Aortic regurgitation has a recognised association with the following:**

A   Reiter's syndrome
B   methysergide therapy
C   polymyalgia rheumatica
D   systemic lupus erythematosus
E   ankylosing spondylitis

Your answers: A.......B.......C.......D.......E.......

13 **In Addisonian pernicious anaemia**

   A   weight loss and fever are recognised presenting features
   B   psychosis and dementia may respond to treatment with vitamin B_{12}
   C   there is a decreased red cell survival accompanied by increased erythropoietic activity which is largely ineffective
   D   serum folate levels are normal or high
   E   a leukoerythroblastic blood picture can occur at presentation

Your answers: A.......B.......C.......D.......E.......

14 **Antagonists at β-adrenoceptors commonly produce**

   A   cold extremities
   B   delayed recovery from hypoglycaemia
   C   enhancement of physiological tremor
   D   nightmares
   E   proliferation of submucosal tissues

Your answers: A.......B.......C.......D.......E.......

15 **The following are true of delirium tremens:**

   A   it occurs in the setting of clear consciousness
   B   there is loss of recent memory
   C   auditory hallucinations often occur
   D   usually starts 48 hours after admission to hospital
   E   about 30% develop Korsakoff's psychosis

Your answers: A.......B.......C.......D.......E.......

16 **Hyperprolactinaemia is a recognised complication of**

   A   thyrotoxicosis
   B   acromegaly
   C   treatment with methyldopa
   D   treatment with allopurinol
   E   hypothyroidism

Your answers: A.......B.......C.......D.......E.......

(17) **Fundus oculi changes are a feature of**

A toxoplasmosis
B cor pulmonale
C Marfan's syndrome
D chloroquine therapy
E aortic arch obstruction (pulseless disease)

Your answers: A.......B.......C.......D.......E.......

(18) **Patients with Klinefelter's syndrome may have**

A abnormal tallness
B gynaecomastia
C mental retardation
D positive buccal smear with 45 chromosomes
E high urinary gonadotrophins

Your answers: A.......B.......C.......D.......E.......

(19) **The neurotransmitter acetylcholine**

A is released at all preganglionic neurones
B is released from neurones which innervate blood vessels in skeletal muscle
C is released from neurones supplying sweat glands
D has the same action on smooth muscle as muscarine
E requires pseudocholinesterase for its inactivation at nerve endings

Your answers: A.......B.......C.......D.......E.......

(20) **The following are recognised associations of fibrosing alveolitis:**

A renal tubular acidosis
B dermatomyositis
C diabetes mellitus
D atrial myxoma
E cranial arteritis

Your answers: A.......B.......C.......D.......E.......

21 **The following conditions are known to give positive tests for rheumatoid factor:**

A   sarcoidosis
B   sub-acute bacterial endocarditis
C   psoriatic arthritis
D   systemic sclerosis
E   chronic liver disease

Your answers: A.......B.......C.......D.......E.......

22 **The following are features of unilateral renal artery stenosis:**

A   hypokalaemic alkalosis
B   renal glycosuria
C   normochromic, normocytic anaemia
D   treatment with Captopril results in a rise in blood urea
E   increased concentration of radiographic contrast on the contralateral side

Your answers: A.......B.......C.......D.......E.......

23 **Regional enteritis**

A   may form fistulous communications to other structures
B   is characterised by exacerbations and remissions
C   may cause narrowing of small intestine
D   is limited to the small bowel
E   may cause steatorrhoea

Your answers: A.......B.......C.......D.......E.......

24 **Thalassaemia major**

A   is a cause of neonatal jaundice
B   is a cause of short stature
C   results in a shortened life-span
D   is a genetic recessive condition
E   results in a bossed forehead

Your answers: A.......B.......C.......D.......E.......

25 **Suspected risk factors other than hypertension for cerebrovascular disease include**

A   diabetes mellitus
B   anaemia
C   oral contraceptives
D   alcholism
E   ischaemic heart disease

Your answers: A.......B.......C.......D.......E.......

26 **Recognised physical signs of mitral regurgitation include**

A   loud first heart sound
B   rumbling diastolic murmur at the apex
C   third heart sound
D   left parasternal pulsation in the absence of right ventricular hypertrophy
E   reversed splitting of the second sound

Your answers: A.......B.......C.......D.......E.......

27 **Cheyne-Stokes breathing is a feature of**

A   uraemia
B   head injury
C   meningitis
D   diabetic coma
E   left ventricular failure

Your answers: A.......B.......C.......D.......E.......

28 **The following statements are true:**

A   ferritin is a better indication of iron stores in secondary anemia than serum iron
B   an iron deficiency blood picture is produced by Thalassemia minor
C   splenomegaly is found in a third of patients with iron deficiency
D   dietary deficiency is the commonest cause of iron deficiency anemia in the UK
E   haemochromatosis may present with ketosis and slaty pigmentation

Your answers: A.......B.......C.......D.......E.......

29 **Minoxidil**

    A   causes arteriolar vasodilatation
    B   accumulates dangerously in renal failure
    C   should not be combined with methyldopa
    D   increases growth of body hair
    E   causes flattening or inversion of the T-wave on the ECG

Your answers: A.......B.......C.......D.......E.......

30 **The following conditions are associated with endogenous depression:**

    A   carcinoma of the pancreas
    B   infectious mononucleosis
    C   temporal lobe epilepsy
    D   acute myocardial infarction
    E   Huntingdon's chorea

Your answers: A.......B.......C.......D.......E.......

31 **The following are recognised causes of permanent cranial diabetes insipidus:**

    A   craniopharyngioma
    B   untreated pituitary adenoma
    C   histiocytosis
    D   sarcoidosis
    E   destruction of posterior lobe of pituitary

Your answers: A.......B.......C.......D.......E.......

32 **The vertebral artery**

    A   is a branch of the lst part of the subclavian artery
    B   enters the costotransverse foramen of the 7th cervical vertebra
    C   enters the skull through the foramen ovale
    D   gives rise to the anterior inferior cerebellar artery
    E   unites with the opposite vertebral artery at the lower border of the pons to form the basilar artery

Your answers: A.......B.......C.......D.......E.......

33 Alopecia areata is

A   preceded by emotional or physical trauma (eg bereavements, divorce, traffic accidents) in at least 80% of cases
B   a recognised association of Down's syndrome
C   a scarring process with permanent loss of follicles
D   pruritic and occasionally painful
E   confined to the scalp hairs

Your answers: A.......B.......C.......D.......E.......

34 The following are features of infection with mumps virus:

A   meningo-encephalitis is a rare complication
B   encephalitis when it occurs always follows a parotitis
C   oophoritis is a well known complication
D   can cause sterility in the adult male
E   pancreatitis is a common complication in adults and children

Your answers: A.......B.......C.......D.......E.......

35 Polymyalgia rheumatica characteristically

A   is associated with raised serum creatinine phosphokinase (CPK) levels
B   affects the shoulder girdles
C   is associated with morning stiffness
D   causes proximal muscle weakness
E   is readily diagnosed by muscle biopsy

Your answers: A.......B.......C.......D.......E.......

36 Membranous glomerulonephritis

A   commonly presents with hypertension
B   responds to steroid therapy
C   is associated with IgG containing immune complexes in the subendothelial portion of the basement membrane
D   can go into spontaneous remission
E   is associated with lung cancer

Your answers: A.......B.......C.......D.......E.......

37 **Marked elevation of serum gastrin levels are found**

A   in Zollinger-Ellison syndrome
B   in duodenal ulcer
C   in pernicious anaemia
D   in gastric ulcer
E   after massive resection of the small bowel

Your answers: A.......B.......C.......D.......E.......

38 **Complications of bacterial meningitis in children include**

A   deafness
B   hydrocephalus
C   epilepsy
D   intellectual retardation
E   cerebral palsy

Your answers: A.......B.......C.......D.......E.......

39 **Polymorphonuclear leucocytosis in CSF is recognised as occurring in**

A   tuberculous meningitis
B   pyogenic meningitis
C   acute postinfective polyneuropathy
D   carcinomatous meningitis
E   disseminated sclerosis

Your answers: A.......B.......C.......D.......E.......

40 **Recognized features of digoxin toxicity include**

A   weight loss
B   unilateral gynaecomastia
C   diplopia
D   ventricular fibrillation
E   delirium

Your answers: A.......B.......C.......D.......E.......

41 **The following dusts are highly fibrogenic to the lung:**

A   silica
B   iron oxide
C   tungsten carbide
D   aluminium
E   tin

Your answers: A.......B.......C.......D.......E.......

42 **In the non-Hodgkin lymphomas**

A   most nodular lymphomas have a good prognosis
B   histiocytic lymphomas comprise 10% of total
C   bone lytic lesions are commonly produced
D   amyloid is a complication
E   B cell surface markers are usually present

Your answers: A.......B.......C.......D.......E.......

43 **Prednisolone in high dosage**

A   abolishes the diurnal variation in cortisol production
B   has little effect on the mean concentration of plasma cortisol
C   increases lymphocyte production
D   lowers the seizure threshold
E   precipitates acute psychotic states

Your answers: A.......B.......C.......D.......E.......

44 **Neurofibromatosis may be associated with**

A   optic atrophy
B   paroxysmal hypertension
C   albuminuria
D   deafness
E   osteosclerosis tibiae

Your answers: A.......B.......C.......D.......E.......

45 Statistical Tests - which of the following are correct?

A   in a chi-squared test the expected frequencies must all be greater than 5
B   an unpaired t-test would be used to compare pulse rates before and after activity
C   a non-parametric test must be used if the data have a normal or Gaussian distribution
D   the Pearson correlation coefficient is a measure of linear association
E   the non-parametric Mann-Whitney U-test is equivalent to the paired t-test

Your answers: A.......B.......C.......D.......E.......

46 Characteristic features of acute falciparum malaria include

A   splenomegaly
B   rigors every 72 hours
C   eosinophilia
D   renal failure
E   recurrence of symptoms after one year in untreated survivors

Your answers: A.......B.......C.......D.......E.......

47 The following statements are true regarding hypothermia in the elderly:

A   in most cases it is due to either hypothyroidism or hypopituitarism
B   it may be caused by chlorpromazine
C   it is associated with post mortem evidence of pancreatitis
D   it is treated by rapid warming and vasodilatory drugs
E   it can be ascribed to hypothyroidism if there is delayed relaxation

Your answers: A.......B.......C.......D.......E.......

48 A patient complains of numbness of hands and feet 10 years after thyroidectomy. The following support diagnosis of hypoparathyroidism:

A   calcification of the basal ganglia
B   macrocytic anaemia
C   cataract formation
D   low plasma phosphate
E   high alkaline phosphatase

Your answers: A.......B.......C.......D.......E.......

49 **The following statements are true of suicide:**

A it is commoner in females
B there has been a marked rise in incidence in recent years
C it occurs most commonly in the spring
D self-poisoning is the method employed in 90% cases
E it is commoner in the younger age group

Your answers: A.......B.......C.......D.......E.......

50 **The following statements are true:**

A complement is an IgM immunoglobulin
B the classical pathway of complement activation is initiated by antigen-antibody complexes
C C_3 convertase is generated solely by the alternative pathway
D hereditary angio-oedema is associated with complement deficiency
E complement is necesary for the agglutination of red cells

Your answers: A.......B.......C.......D.......E.......

51 **The following are features of Legionnaires' disease:**

A it has a mortality of 15-20% in all cases
B it has an attack rate of less than 5%
C it is caused by a gram negative bacillus
D fatal cases usually have renal failure
E patients who recover may have a long term lung damage from the disease

Your answers: A.......B.......C.......D.......E.......

52 **The following are recognized features of rheumatoid disease**

A solitary granuloma of lung
B osteogenic sarcoma
C crescentic glomerulonephritis
D iritis
E pleural effusion

Your answers: A.......B.......C.......D.......E.......

53 **In lymphogranuloma venereum**

    A   the causative organism is *Chlamydia trachomatis*
    B   lesions are confined to the genital area
    C   the primary lesion is characteristically transient
    D   serological tests are of no diagnostic value
    E   tetracycline is the treatment of choice

Your answers: A.......B.......C.......D.......E.......

54 **Ascites is a feature of**

    A   acute pericarditis
    B   tuberculous peritonitis
    C   Meigs's syndrome
    D   metastatic carcinoma
    E   alcoholic liver disease

Your answers: A.......B.......C.......D.......E.......

55 **Malabsorption in infancy may be due to**

    A   gluten enteropathy
    B   threadworm infestation
    C   iron deficiency
    D   lactase deficiency
    E   abdominal radiotherapy

Your answers: A.......B.......C.......D.......E.......

56 **Left atrial myxoma may be associated with the following features:**

    A   signs suggesting mitral stenosis
    B   syncope
    C   acute pulmonary oedema
    D   cerebrovascular accident
    E   increased erythrocyte sedimentation rate

Your answers: A.......B.......C.......D.......E.......

57 **The following are signs of respiratory failure:**

A   warm hands
B   small volume pulse
C   flapping tremor
D   papilloedema
E   altered level of consciousness

Your answers: A.......B.......C.......D.......E.......

58 **The following are features of myelomatosis:**

A   leg ulcers
B   amyloidosis
C   lymphadenopathy
D   renal tubular defects
E   pathological fractures

Your answers: A.......B.......C.......D.......E.......

59 **Sulphasalazine**

A   absorption is virtually complete
B   is effective by enema in inflammatory bowel disease
C   inhibits prostaglandin synthesis
D   has caused haemolytic anaemia
E   reduces fertility

Your answers: A.......B.......C.......D.......E.......

60 **The following statements are true:**

A   the ulnar nerve supplies the majority of flexor muscles in the forearm
B   the ulnar nerve supplies the majority of the intrinsic muscles of the hand
C   the median nerve supplies the hypothenar muscles
D   the radial nerve supplies the dorsal interossei
E   the radial nerve supplies the majority of the extensor muscles in the forearm

Your answers: A.......B.......C.......D.......E.......

END OF EXAM 2

Go over your answers until your time is up. Answers and explanations are on page 88.

Time allowed 2½ hours

1 **Vesicles are characteristic in**

A   exfoliative dermatitis
B   erythema multiforme
C   dermatitis herpetiformis
D   porphyria cutanea tarda
E   Stevens-Johnson syndrome

Your answers: A.......B. ..C.. ...D.......E...

2 **In thyroid cancer**

A   hyperthyroidism is often present
B   anaplastic lesions typically occur in the young
C   there is characteristically a 'hot nodule' on radioisotope scanning of the thyroid gland
D   bone metastases are exceptional
E   the papillary type carries a better prognosis than the follicular type

Your answers: A. ..B. ..C.......D. ...E... ..

3 **Automosal dominance is exemplified in**

A   haemophilia
B   arachnodactyly
C   polyposis coli
D   cystinuria
E   dystrophia myotonica

Your answers: A. ..B.......C.. ..D.......E... ..

4 **Renal papillary necrosis is a recognised complication of**

A   medullary sponge kidney
B   sickle cell anaemia
C   acute pancreatitis
D   diabetes mellitus
E   sulphonamide nephrotoxicity

Your answers: A.....B.....C.......D.......E.

5 **Diverticular disease of the colon**

   A   can give heavy rectal bleeding
   B   often presents with abdominal pain
   C   may give rise to perianal fistulae
   D   the diverticula occur on the side of the colon opposite the mesentery
   E   is rarely found in patients with recto-sigmoid cancer

Your answers: A.. ..B... ..C....D.......E.. ..

6 **In disseminated sclerosis, plaques of demyelination characteristically occur in the**

   A   cervical segments of the spinal cord
   B   anterior horn cells
   C   optic nerves
   D   periaqueductal region of the midbrain
   E   posterior nerve roots

Your answers: A. ..B.......C.......D.: ...E.. ...

7 **Infective endocarditis**

   A   is a recognised cause of glomerulonephritis
   B   when due to *Streptococcus faecalis* should be treated with intravenous benzyl penicillin alone
   C   is a recognised complication of brucellosis
   D   may be excluded as a diagnosis if splenomegaly is absent
   E   may follow sigmoidoscopy

Your answers: A.......B.....C... .D. ...E. ...

8 *Pneumocystis carinii* **infection**

   A   occurs only in the immunosuppressed
   B   responds to treatment with co-trimoxazole (Septrin)
   C   can usually be diagnosed by examination of the sputum
   D   may produce gaseous cysts in the wall of the colon
   E   in the lung is frequently accompanied by cytomegalovirus infection

Your answers: A. .B. ..C .D.. ...E.. .

9 **In polycythaemia rubra vera**

A generalised pruritus is typically worse after a hot bath
B a low MCV is a recognised complication
C gout is a recognised complication
D the diagnostic value of raised leucocyte alkaline phosphatase is limited
E splenomegaly is found in 75% of cases

Your answers: A.. ....B.. ...C.. ...D.......E.. ..

10 **Slow acetylators are more prone to the following adverse drug effect:**

A haemolysis with methyldopa
B hepatitis with isoniazid
C nausea and vomiting with sulphasalazine
D peripheral neuropathy with isoniazid
E systemic lupus syndrome with hydralazine

Your answers: A... .B... ..C.. ...D...\ ..E.......

11 **The following statements are true of bronchiolitis:**

A up to 50% of patients continue to wheeze after recovery
B the typical pathogen is para influenza virus
C corticosteroid therapy is beneficial
D tachypnoea is invariable
E air-trapping is normally present

Your answers: A.(..B... ..C... ..D.. ...E.......

12 **In the leg**

A spasticity in a patient with hemiplegia leads to eversion of the foot
B the lateral popliteal (common peroneal) nerve passes lateral to the neck of the fibula
C foot drop is due to paralysis of the femoral nerve
D the long saphenous vein lies 2.5cm in front of the medial malleolus
E the posterior tibial artery is normally felt behind the medial malleolus

Your answers: A.......B.:.....C.. ..D..: ..E.. ..

(13) The following are true of hysteria:

A it tends to occur in persons of a previously normal personality
B "la belle indifference" is invariably present
C stupor in a young person is more often due to schizophrenia than to hysteria
D characteristically appears for the first time in middle age
E the hysteric usually looks physically ill

Your answers: A.......B.......C.......D.......E.. ....

(14) In the treatment of rheumatoid arthritis

A the symptomatic benefit from non-steroid anti-inflammatory drugs is associated with a fall in the ESR and the concentration of C-reactive protein
B gold therapy modifies the course of the disease
C some side-effects to D-penicillamine and gold may be predicted on a genetic basis
D plasmaphoresis is helpful treatment
E steroids particularly predispose patients to developing septic arthritis

Your answers: A.. ...B... ...C... .D.... E..

(15) Plasma proteins

A on electrophoresis migrate at different rates to the anode and cathode
B contribute largely to the osmotic pressure of plasma
C concentration falls early in starvation
D are involved in the transport of thyroid, adrenocortical and gonadal hormones
E are responsible for 15% of the buffering capacity of the blood

Your answers: A.. ...B.. .C.......D.. .E.. ..

(16) Which of the following conditions result in enlarged kidneys:

A acute renal failure following hypovolaemic shock
B analgesic nephropathy
C amyloidosis
D chronic glomerulonephritis
E polycystic kidneys

Your answers: A. ..B... ..C. .D. ...E.: ..

17 *Campylobacter jejuni* **(formerly** *Vibrio fetus)*

    A   infection is significantly associated with childhood diarrhoea
    B   infections are treated with ampicillin
    C   is a recognised pathogen in dogs
    D   requires special atmospheric conditions for culture
    E   can be sigmoidoscopically indistinguishable from ulcerative colitis

Your answers: A. ...B.. ..C.......D.......E.. ..

18 **In chronic alcoholism**

    A   delirium tremens may be precipitated by a surgical operation
    B   the cerebellar disturbance characteristically involves the arms and speech and spares the gait
    C   epilepsy is a recognised associated feature
    D   central pontine myelinolysis is a recognised complication
    E   dementia rarely occurs even in long standing cases

Your answers: A... ..B.......C.. ...D.. ..E.. ..

19 **Glyceryl trinitrate**

    A   increases coronary flow in ischaemic heart disease
    B   causes venoconstriction
    C   lowers the arterial blood pressure
    D   can produce methaemoglobinaemia
    E   is effective for only 5 minutes when given sublingually

Your answers: A. ...B.. ..C. ....D.. ...E... .

20 **Legionnaires' disease**

    A   is caused by a small gram negative bacillus
    B   may present with diarrhoea
    C   should be treated with erythromycin
    D   is associated with leucopenia
    E   causes microscopic haematuria in 10% patients

Your answers: A... .B... ..C.. ...D.......E.. .

21 **Bleeding in the following conditions is due to thrombocytopenia:**

A   von Willebrand's disease
B   aspirin poisoning
C   Goodpasture's syndrome
D   oxyphenbutazone therapy
E   scurvy

Your answers: A.......B.......C.......D.......E.......

22 **The risk of intoxication during digoxin treatment is increased by**

A   hypercalcaemia
B   hyperkalaemia
C   hypoalbuminaemia
D   hypokalaemia
E   hypomagnesaemia

Your answers: A.......B.......C.......D.......E.......

23 **In rheumatoid arthritis**

A   synovial fluid cells are predominantly polymorphonuclear
B   rheumatoid factors are autoantibodies against altered IgM
C   patients with positive rheumatoid factor have subcutaneous rheumatoid nodules
D   50% of cases with digital infarcts have positive rheumatoid factor
E   knee involvement can mimic deep calf vein thrombosis

Your answers: A.......B.......C.......D.......E.......

24 **The following are features of *Schistosoma haematobium*:**

A   pruritus
B   glomerulonephritis
C   hydronephrosis
D   successful response to trivalent arsenical drugs
E   eosinophilia

Your answers: A.......B.......C.......D.......E.......

25 **The following are true of arterioslerotic dementia:**

A it has the same age distribution as senile dementia
B the condition runs a steadily progressive course
C emotional lability is common
D insight tends to be retained
E depression is uncommon

Your answers: A ...B.......C.. ...D ...E.. ...

26 **In diabetic ketoacidaemic coma**

A intraocular pressure is raised
B the acidaemia should be rapidly corrected with 8.4% sodium bicarbonate intravenously
C severe abdominal pain and vomiting at the onset suggest that the patient has acute pancreatitis
D the depth of coma is directly related to the degree of blood glucose elevation present
E intravenous infusion of tolbutamide forms a satisfactory alternative to treatment with insulin

Your answers: A.. :..B. ...C.. ...D..'....E.. ...

27 **The affinity of haemoglobin for oxygen is**

A decreased by alkalosis
B decreased by increasing body temperature
C increased by increasing concentrations of 2, 3 diphosphoglycerate
D decreased by serotonin
E decreased by hypoxia

Your answers: A.......B.......C.......D.......E.......

28 **The following statements about nephrotic syndrome are true:**

A the prognosis in children is poor compared with that in adults
B non-selective proteinuria gives a better prognosis
C it increases susceptibility to infection
D hypercholesterolaemia is invariably present
E it can occur after heavy metal poisoning

Your answers: A. ...B.. ...C. ..D.......E... ...

29 **Alphafoetoprotein**

A   is an antibody
B   can be detected with greater sensitivity by immune electrophoresis than by radioimmunoassay
C   is greatly raised in a pregnancy associated with anencephaly
D   is found more often and in high titres in the more undifferentiated hepatomas
E   when detected in a patient with liver disease always indicates the presence of a hepatoma

Your answers: A.......B........C.. ..D.. ..E.. .

30 **The following statements regarding polyneuropathy are correct:**

A   world-wide the commonest cause of polyneuropathy is leprosy
B   in post-infective polyneuritis patchy demyelination is the predominant pathological finding
C   renal transplantation has no effect on uraemic neuropathy
D   the neuropathy associated with isoniazid therapy may be prevented by the administration of vitamin C
E   diabetic femoral neuropathy is usually associated with an acute painless onset of wasting and weakness of the quadriceps femoris

Your answers: A.. .B.......C.. .D... .E .....

31 **A third heart sound in a 45 year old man**

A   is a sign of heart disease
B   excludes significant mitral stenosis
C   could be due to tricuspid regurgitation
D   is a feature of constrictive pericarditis
E   could indicate hypertensive heart disease

Your answers: A. ..B.. ...C. ..D.......E... .

32 **The diagnosis of farmers' lung is supported by a**

A   history of exposure to mouldy hay
B   reduced diffusion capacity
C   cough with profuse expectoration
D   pronounced eosinophilia
E   seasonal incidence May to July

Your answers: A.. ..B.......C... ..D.......E.......

33 The risk of pregnancy despite combined contraceptive steroid usage is increased by concurrent treatment with

    A   diazepam
    B   isoniazid
    C   phenobarbitone
    D   phenytoin
    E   rifampicin

Your answers: A.......Ρ ...C.. ..D. ..E. ..

34 Intracranial calcification may be a feature of

    A   Huntingdon's chorea
    B   taboparesis
    C   tuberculoma
    D   subdural haematoma
    E   toxoplasmosis

Your answers: A. ..B.......C.. ..D. ..E. ..

35 The following statements are true of cystic fibrosis:

    A   inheritance is autosomal dominant
    B   respiratory failure is the usual cause of death
    C   anaemia is frequently found
    D   males are sterile
    E   nasal polyps are significantly associated

Your answers: A... ..B. .C ..D.. ..E. ..

36 Section 29 of the Mental Health Act (1959)

    A   allows for compulsory detention for a period of 48 hours
    B   requires the authorization of two Medical Practitioners
    C   requires the authorization of a Psychiatrist
    D   a Social Worker may apply for the patient's admission
    E   relatives may not apply for the patient's admission

Your answers: A.......B.......C.......D.......E.......

(37) Hirsutism in females

A when idiopathic, is associated with normal plasma testerone levels
B can be caused by phenytoin
C when ovarian in origin, is most commonly due to arrhenoblastoma
D is a presenting symptom of hyperprolactinaemia
E may be due to congenital adrenal hyperplasia

Your answers: A.......B.......C.....D.......E...

(38) Characteristic features of trichinosis include

A eosinophilia
B periorbital oedema
C petechial rash
D muscle tenderness
E subungual haemorrhages

Your answers: A.....B.....C.......D....E......

(39) Carpal tunnel syndrome is associated with

A Cushing's syndrome
B rheumatoid arthritis
C primary amyloidosis
D myxoedema
E systemic lupus erythematosus

Your answers: A.......B.....C.....D....E..

(40) In cancer of the oesophagus

A the commonest site is the middle third of the oesophagus
B when occuring at the gastro-oesophageal level is equally likely to be an adenocarcinoma as squamous epithelial
C is a complication of Barrett's oesophagus
D chest pain is a late symptom
E is a complication of coeliac disease

Your answers: A.....B.......C......D....E.....

41 A lesion confined to one side of the pons would be expected to produce

A ipsilateral hemianaesthesia
B contralateral hemiplegia
C ipsilateral wasting of the tongue
D diplopia
E nystagmus

Your answers: A.... ..B.. ..C...' .D.... ..E... ..

42 The following statements apply to bronchial carcinoma:

A sputum cytology produces 30% false positive results
B sputum cytology is of value in pulmonary metastases
C confusion indicates cerebral metastases
D the incidence in females is rising
E haemoptysis suggests a poor prognosis

Your answers: A.......B... .C.. ..D..: .E.(.

43 Splenectomy

A results in increased incidence of pneumococcal septicemia
B is a valuable diagnostic procedure in non-Hodgkin lymphoma
C produces blood film appearance of acanthocytes and Howell Jolly bodies
D produces appearances which are also occasionally seen in coeliac disease in the absence of surgery
E produces almost invariable remission in hereditary spherocytosis

Your answers: A. ..B.(.C(..D.......E.. ..

44 The risk of gastrointestinal bleeding during warfarin treatment is increased by concurrent administration of

A aspirin
B diazepam
C paracetamol
D phenobarbitone
E phenylbutazone

Your answers: A.. .B... .C.(..D.(.E... .

45 **The following statements are true of whooping cough:**

A   absolute lymphocytosis occurs
B   encephalopathy may occur
C   the disease may present without cough history
D   cough suppressants are beneficial
E   subconjunctival haemorrhage occurs

Your answers: A.. ..B.... ..C.. ..D.. .E.. ..

46 **bilirubin metabolism**

A   unconjugated bilirubin is all derived from the breakdown of haemoglobin by the reticulo-endothelial system
B   conjugation by microsomes in the smooth endoplasmic reticulum can be increased by administration of phenobarbitone
C   novobiocin jaundice is due to competitive inhibition of glucuronyl transferase
D   methyltestosterone jaundice is due to competitive inhibition of glucuronyl transferase
E   bilirubin in the gut lumen is hydrolysed to unconjugated bilirubin prior to reduction to urobilinogen

Your answers: A.......B... ..C.......D.......E.. .

47 **The following neurological signs are common findings in the elderly and are of little or no pathological significance:**

A   absent superficial abdominal reflexes
B   bilateral absence of ankle reflexes
C   absent pupillary response to light
D   absent sensation to vibration at the ankles
E   positive grasp reflex

Your answers: A... ..B.... C... .D... ..E... .

48 **The following are features of Cushing's syndrome**

A   hypertension
B   psychiatric symptomatology
C   short stature in children
D   hirsutes
E   polycythaemia

Your answers: A.. ..B... ..C... ..D... .E..

49 **Visual impairment results from direct infection of the eye in**

   A onchocerciasis
   B toxocariasis
   C trachoma
   D toxoplasmosis
   E Chaga's disease

Your answers: A.. ...B.. ....C.......D......E.. ...

50 **In systemic sclerosis**

   A subcutaneous calcification (calcinosis) is associated with a good prognosis
   B D-penicillamine influences the progression of the disease
   C avoidance of exposure to cold is important
   D oesophageal involvement is related to an adverse prognosis
   E the 10-year survival rate is approximately 10%

Your answers: A. ..B.. ..C.. ...D... ..E.......

51 **In chronic renal failure due to glomerulo-nephritis, the following are reduced in the serum:**

   A pH
   B bicarbonate
   C phosphate
   D calcium
   E creatinine

Your answers: A. ..B.......C. ...D.. ...E.. :.

52 **In Parkinson's disease**

   A the concentration of dopamine in the substantia nigra is decreased
   B the onset of symptoms is typically before the age of 40
   C there is characteristically a positive family history
   D ankle clonus is characteristic
   E chlorpromazine will abolish the tremor

Your answers: A ..B. ..C.. ...D.......E(

53 **Causes of atrial fibrillation include**

A   hyperthyroidism
B   recent myocardial infarction
C   anxiety
D   cardiac surgery
E   ventricular septal defect

Your answers: A.. ...B... ..C.. ...D.......E. ..

54 **The sciatic nerve**

A   divides into tibial and common peroneal nerves at a variable level in the lower limb
B   lies under cover of gluteus maximus midway between the greater trochanter and the ischial tuberosity
C   is derived from the ventral rami of the L4, 5 and S1, 2 and 3 spinal nerves
D   supplies the gluteal muscles
E   is the main nerve supplying the adductor magnus

Your answers: A.......B.......C.......D.. .E...

55 **The following statements concerning sarcoidosis are true:**

A   erythema nodosum usually indicates a benign course
B   hypercalcaemia indicates parathyroid involvement
C   cortiscosteroid therapy is indicated if there is posterior uveitis
D   the value of the Kveim test is limited because of many false positives
E   leucocytosis is nearly always present

Your answers: A.. ....B... ..C.. ,D.. E... .

56 **During treatment of acute lymphoblastic leukaemia in children there is serious hazard from**

A   chicken pox
B   measles
C   cytomegalovirus infection
D   injection of live poliomyelitis vaccine
E   injection of diphtheria toxoid

Your answers: A.. ..B.......C.. ...D.. .E.......

57 **The therapeutic efficacy of the first drug is greater than that of the second:**

A   bumetanide, frusemide
B   frusemide, bendrofluazide
C   indomethacin, aspirin
D   morphine, methadone
E   pethidine, codeine

Your answers: A.......B.. .C.... ..D.......E... .

58 **The following are features of Down's syndrome:**

A   cataract
B   umbilical hernia
C   atresia of the foregut
D   Brushfield's spots
E   asthma

Your answers: A.. ..B.......C... ..D.. ..E......

59 **Distributions - which of the following statements are correct:**

A   the mean equals the variance in the Poisson Distribution
B   the sample mean, median and mode have the same value for normally distributed data
C   if the probability of an event is 0.1 for a binomial variable then the probability of the event not occurring is -0.1
D   for large sample sizes, the shapes of the Normal, Binomial and Poisson distributions are similar
E   in positively skewed data the median is greater than the mode

Your answers: A.......B.' .C.......D.. ..E..

60 **Characteristic features of thromboembolic or primary pulmonary hypertension include**

A   dominant S wave in ECG lead V_1
B   large A wave in jugular venous pulse
C   exertional dyspnoea
D   angina
E   finger clubbing

Correct 172
Wrong 46
Total 126 = 42%
300

Your answers: A. ..B. ..C......D. ..E.. ..

END OF EXAM 3

Go over your answers until your time is up. Answers and explanations are on page 99.

PRACTICE EXAM 4

Time allowed: 2½ hours

1 **The following therapies provide relief from a severe attack of bronchial asthma within minutes:**

A intravenous aminophylline
B intravenous hydrocortisone
C ipratropium by aerosol
D intravenous salbutamol
E terbutaline respirator solution delivered by intermittent positive pressure ventilation

Your answers: A... B.. ..C.. ...D. ...E.. ...

2 **In acute myeloid leukaemia in adults**

A full haematological remission can be induced in the majority of patients by appropriate chemotherapy
B if remission is induced the expected survival is 5 to 6 years
C survival can be prolonged by immunotherapy with irradiated acute myeloid leukaemia blast cells
D bone marrow transplantation requires prior destruction of the recipient's marrow and immune system with chemotherapy and irradiation
E bone marrow transplantation may be followed by fatal graft - versus - host disease

Your answers: A.. ...B... .C.. ...D. ....E. ...

3 **The femoral nerve supplies**

A the gluteus minimus muscle
B the rectus femoris muscle
C the skin over the lateral malleolus
D the iliacus muscle
E the ankle joint

Your answers: A..'....B.. ....C. ..D.. ...E.. ...

4 **Miliary calcification of the lungs on X-ray occurs in**

A chalk dust inhalation
B chicken pox
C asbestosis
D histoplasmosis
E sarcoidosis

Your answers: A.......B.......C......D.....E. ..

5) **In hypertrophic obstructive cardiomyopathy (HOCM)**

A   atrial fibrillation indicates a poor prognosis
B   the characteristic murmur is loudest in the aortic area
C   propranolol therapy prevents the complication of sudden death
D   trinitrin reduces outflow obstruction
E   there are characteristic echocardiographic findings

Your answers: A. .B. ..C. ..D.. ....E......

6) **Which of the following are true of motor neurone disease:**

A   it is commoner in men than women
B   root pain is common
C   sphincters are involved late in the disease
D   myotonia is a feature
E   fasciculation of muscle occurs

Your answers: A. ....B... ..C......D......E.. ..

7) **The following are recognised features of hiatus hernia:**

A   anorexia
B   anaemia
C   morning vomiting
D   skin pigmentation
E   aggravation of symptoms during pregnancy

Your answers: A.. ..B.. ..C.......D. ..E.. ...

8) **Characteristic associations of polyarteritis nodosa include**

A   renal involvement in about 80% of cases
B   aneurysm formation affecting medium sized arteries
C   eosinophilia
D   positive HBsAg
E   abnormal C_3 complement level

Your answers: A.......B.....C.. ..D... ..E... .

9 **Joint pain and swelling occur in**

    A   thrombocytopenic purpura
    B   haemophilia
    C   acute post-streptococcal glomerulonephritis
    D   sarcoidosis
    E   gonorrhoea

Your answers: A.......B.......C.. ...D.. ....E... ...

10 **A defective X chromosome occurs in**

    A   haemophilia
    B   Duchenne muscular dystrophy
    C   congenital pyloric stenosis
    D   Huntingdon's chorea
    E   cystic fibrosis of the pancreas

Your answers: A.....B.. ...C......D. ...E ....

11 **In phaeochromocytoma**

    A   50% of the tumours are extra adrenal in location
    B   postural hypotension is a recognised finding
    C   retroperitoneal insufflation of carbon dioxide is the most effective method of localising the tumour
    D   there is a recognised association with medullary carcinoma of the thyroid
    E   beta adrenoceptor blocking drugs alone are effective in controlling hypertensive episodes preoperatively

Your answers: A.....B.......C. ..D. ...E.. ..

12 **In a 70 year old man with tremor of the upper limbs, essential tremor rather than Parkinsonism is more likely to be the cause if**

    A   the tremor is worst at rest
    B   alcohol increases the tremor
    C   propanolol reduces the tremor
    D   there is no akinesia or rigidity
    E   there is no family history of tremor

Your answers: A. ...B.. ..C. ..D.. ...E.. .

13 **Right coronary artery**

A lies in the groove between the right atrium and right ventricle
B typically supplies the inferior aspect of the left ventricle
C typically gives rise to the artery to the A-V node
D gives rise to the left marginal branch
E arises from the right posterior aortic sinus

Your answers: A... ..B. ...C. ...D.. ..E.......

14 **Captopril**

A accumulates in renal failure
B causes potassium depletion
C inhibits angiotensin converting enzyme
D is contraindicated in severe heart failure
E reduces blood pressure in normotensive individuals

Your answers: A. ...B.. ..C. ....D......E.... .

15 **Cold agglutinins**

A are found regularly in *Mycoplasma pneumoniae*
B may produce acute haemolysis in infectious mononucleosis
C in high titre frequently produce Raynaud's phenomenon
D commonly produce transfusion reactions
E are a complication of gonococcal infection

Your answers: A... ..B... .C.... .D.......E..

16 **Diffuse interstitial fibrosis in the early stage is characterised by**

A cyanosis at rest
B reduced vital capacity
C reduced FEV_1/FVC ratio
D bilateral reticular shadowing on chest X-ray
E reduced pulmonary diffusing capacity

Your answers: A.. ..B.! ..C.. ..D.. ...E. ..

(17) **The mitral diastolic murmur of Austin Flint**

A is associated with a loud first heart sound
B is an early sign of aortic regurgitation
C can be distinguished from the murmur of mitral stenosis by absence of presystolic accentuation
D is due to partial closure of the posterior leaflet of the mitral valve
E does not occur in aortic incompetence secondary to an aortitis

Your answers: A. ...B.. ..C.. ..D... .E.... .

(18) **In migrainous neuralgia (Cluster headache)**

A the attacks tend to occur at night
B the pain is always unilateral
C the pain commonly lasts up to 12 hours
D there may be ptosis on the affected side
E the attacks may be precipitated by alcohol

Your answers: A.. ..B.. ..C. ...D.......E.. ..

(19) **The following statements are true of infant feeding:**

A in human milk the predominant immunoglobulin is IgM
B a woman can produce two litres of milk per day
C babies consume approximately 250 ml/Kg/day
D human milk provides less vitamin D than the recommended daily amount
E breast feeding prevents atopic conditions

Your answers: A.. ..B.... ..C.... D. ..E.. ..

(20) **Renal failure in multiple myeloma is associated with the following:**

A amyloidosis
B hyperuricaemia
C intravenous pyelography
D glomerular destruction by precipitation of kappa and lambda light chains in Bowman's space
E hypercalcaemia

Your answers: A.. ..B.. ....D. ..E... .

Correct 67
Wrong 18
─────
49 /.

21 Systemic lupus erythematosus

A is about twice as common in women than men
B is a cause of false positive tests for syphilis
C is not significantly associated with oral and nasal ulceration
D can only be diagnosed if circulating immune complexes are present
E usually causes a lymphocytosis

Your answers: A.. ..B.. ..C.......D. ..E.. ..

22 In the differential diagnosis of fever in a 35 year old man

A an ESR of 100 mm/hour is highly suggestive of multiple myeloma
B an ESR of 100 mm/hour is highly suggestive of polymyalgia rheumatica
C a white cell count over 14,000/mm³ makes brucellosis unlikely
D a negative skin test for tuberculosis makes this diagnosis unlikely
E a packed cell volume of 0.52 suggests the need for renal radiology

Your answers: A.. ...B. ...C. ..D.. ..E... .

23 Actions of glucagon include

A glycogenolysis in the liver
B inhibition of insulin secretion
C gluconeogenesis in the liver
D inhibition of adenyl cyclase
E a positive inotropic effect on the heart

Your answers: A.. ..B.. ..C.. ..D.......E. ..

24 The following statements are true of tricyclic antidepressants:

A they are effective in most patients with reactive depression
B they may be prescribed following acute myocardial infarction
C they produce EEG changes
D they may potentiate the effects of anticoagulants
E they may cause weight gain

Your answers: A.. ..B... C.. ...D... ..E.. ..

25 **The pain of trigeminal neuralgia**

A   is associated with sensory loss in affected division
B   may be triggered by exposure to cold winds
C   rarely affects the first division of the nerve
D   is nearly always unilateral
E   is commoner in males than in females

Your answers: A. ...B. ..C.....D. ...E.. . .

26 **The following are adverse effects observed during therapy of reversible airways obstruction:**

A   bronchospasm on inhalation of sodium cromoglycate powder
B   increased sputum viscosity after parenteral atropine
C   oropharyngeal candidiasis in users of beclomethasone aerosols
D   tremor provoked by intravenous terbutaline
E   vomiting provoked by intravenous aminophylline

Your answers: A.: ...B.......C.. ...D.. .E... .

27 **Paraproteins may sometimes be detected in the serum of patients with**

A   malignant lymphoma
B   scleroderma
C   chronic myeloid leukaemia
D   chronic lymphatic leukaemia
E   Kaposi's sarcoma

Your answers: A.......B... ..C.... .D.. ...E....

28 **In acute respiratory acidosis**

A   the plasma bicarbonate ion concentration rises
B   the plasma hydrogen ion concentration falls
C   the arterial PO_2 is always low
D   the affinity of haemoglobin for oxygen increases
E   minute ventilation is characteristically lower than normal

Your answers: A... .B... ..C.. ..D.. ..E.. ..

29 A 24 year old girl who is asymptomatic presents with a systolic murmur of grade 3/6 intensity, maximal at the pulmonary area. The following would support a diagnosis of a secundum atrial septal defect:

A a mid-diastolic murmur at the left sternal edge
B a chest X-ray showing a small aortic knuckle, prominent pulmonary artery and pulmonary plethora
C wide fixed splitting of the second sound
D pulmonary ejection click
E an electrocardiogram showing right bundle branch block with left axis deviation

Your answers: A.... ..B.. ..C ...D.......E.... ..

30 Epileptic attacks may be precipitated by the following

A viral encephalitis
B hypocalcaemia
C tricyclic antidepressant drugs
D adjusting a television set
E trivial head injuries

Your answers: A... .B... ...C.. ..D... ...E... ...

31 In juvenile arthritis, the following may occur:

A irido-cyclitis
B papular rash
C micrognathia
D positive SCAT test
E femoral condylar hypertrophy

Your answers: A.. ...B.. ..C.. ..D.......E.. ....

32 Presence of gall stones may be associated with the following clinical picture:

A obstructive jaundice
B acute pancreatitis
C haemolytic jaundice
D no symptoms or signs
E an acute abdomen

Your answers: A.. ...B... ..C... ..D... .E.....

33 **Recognized features of generalised osteoarthrosis include**

A Clutton's joints
B Schmorl's nodes
C Heberden's nodes
D Bouchard's nodes
E Romanus lesions

Your answers: A..... .B.. ..C.. ...D.......E ..

34 **The following are features of rabies virus infection:**

A it can be carried by foxes for several weeks
B it can be harmless to small mammals
C it is found only in the brain at autopsy
D fatal infections always make dogs mad
E it can have an incubation period longer than six months

Your answers: A......B.......C.......D.....E... .

35 **The following drugs may raise serum thyroxine:**

A salicylates
B phenytoin
C clofibrate
D oestrogens
E androgens

Your answers: A... .B.. ...C(,.D.: ..E.. ...

36 **The following are associated with dementia:**

A pernicious anaemia
B hypervitaminosis A
C pellagra
D porphyria
E Wilson's disease

Your answers: A.. ...B.. ...C..' ..D.. ...E.. ...

37 Given the following data 1. 1. 2. 3. 3. 4. 4. 4. 5. 13 which of the following are correct:

A   the node is 4
B   the median is 3
C   the mean is 4
D   given the standard deviation is 3. 43 the variance is 6. 86
E   the standard error is the standard deviation divided by the sample size

Your answers: A... ...B.. ..C... ..D.... .E. ....

38 These two agents are incompatible if solutions are mixed:

A   calcium gluconate, sodium bicarbonate
B   morphine, perphenazine
C   phenytoin sodium, dextrose
D   soluble insulin, isophane insulin
E   ticarcillin, gentamicin

Your answers: A... ..B... .C.. .D.... .E.......

39 Disseminated intravascular coagulation

A   is often characterised by neurological presentation
B   produces fragmented red cells
C   produces thrombocytopenia
D   responds to heparin therapy in the majority of cases
E   is characterised by raised fibrin degradation products

Your answers: A.......B.......C. ...D. ..E... ..

40 The following typically appear in the anterior mediastinum:

A   syphilitic aortic aneurysm
B   dermoid
C   thymoma
D   neuroblastoma
E   neurofibroma

Your answers: A... ..B.. ...C.. .D.. ..E. ....

41 **The following statements about subacute infective endocarditis (SABE) are correct:**

A   splinter haemorrhages are due to septic microemboli
B   the condition is a frequent complication of osteum secundum atrial septal defects
C   vegetations may be recognised by echocardiography
D   left atrial myxoma is an important differential diagnosis
E   haematuria is exceptional

Your answers: A... .B. ....C. ...D. ...E. ....

42 **Chorea is a recognized manifestation of**

A   oral contraceptive therapy
B   systemic lupus erythematosus
C   polycythaemia rubra vera
D   myxoedema
E   phenytoin medication

Your answers: A. ...B.......C......D......E.. ...

43 **In childhood asthma**

A   over 90% of patients show exercise-induced bronchoconstriction
B   hypercapnia is the first physiological disturbance in status asthmaticus
C   infants are unresponsive to bronchodilators
D   spontaneous cure occurs before adolescence
E   cough may be the only symptom

Your answers: A.......B.......C.. ...D..: ...E.....

44 **Pseudomembranous colitis**

A   has a characteristic appearance on sigmoidoscopy
B   is a notifiable disease
C   is treated with parenteral vancomycin
D   is characterised by a toxin produced by *Clostridium difficile*
E   can be spread by cross infection

Your answers: A... .B.......C... ..D.. ...E.......

45   Anaemia in chronic renal failure

A   becomes evident when glomerular filtration rate falls below 30 ml/min
B   is reversed by dialysis
C   is least marked in patients with polycystic kidneys
D   is tolerated by most patients because of an increase in red cell 2, 3 diphosphoglycerate (2, 3 DPG)
E   due to iron deficiency is recognised by a low serum iron

Your answers: A.... ...B.. ...C.   ...D. ...E.......

46   Cyclic AMP (adenosine -3, 5-monophosphate)

A   is formed from ATP (adenosine-triphosphate)
B   mediates the effects of many peptide hormones
C   mediates the effects of many steroid hormones
D   acts via activation of plasma kinase
E   is inhibited by caffeine and theophylline

Your answers: A.......B..' ..C.. .:D.. ...E.' ..

47   Which of the following conditions cause unilateral blindness of rapid onset:

A   detachment of retina
B   central retinal artery embolism
C   vitreous haemorrhage
D   retinitis pigmentosa
E   retrobulbar neuritis

Your answers: A.:....B... ..C.'.....D.. ..E... .

48   Puerperal psychosis

A   usually begins after the second week of the puerperium
B   often takes the form of schizophrenia
C   recurrence of puerperal psychosis in subsequent pregnancies is the rule
D   the onset is usually insidious
E   the prognosis is usually good

Your answers: A.......B... ..C. ....D. ...E... ..

49   The following statements are true:

A   Marburg virus disease characteristically produces a maculopapular rash against a background of pronounced erythema

B   Lassa fever is an acute febrile disease of man caused by an arbovirus

C   a recognised association of Ebola virus disease is vomiting, abdominal cramps and diarrhoea

D   yellow fever vaccine can be given at the same time as smallpox vaccine

E   louping ill is transmitted via infected mosquitos

Your answers: A.......B.......C.... ..D.......E.......

50   The following associations are correct in pulmonary disease:

A   basal fibrosis and ankylosing spondylitis

B   pleurisy with effusion and Sjogren's syndrome

C   basal pneumonia and systemic sclerosis

D   chylothorax and yellow nails

E   lymphangitis - carcinomatosa and carcinoma of the pancreas

Your answers: A.. .B... ..C....C..D.:. ..E. ...

51   ST depression on ECG may found in

A   digitalis toxicity

B   hypertension

C   hypervitaminosis D

D   chronic pericarditis

E   chronic thiazide administration

Your answers: A.. .B.. ..C.......D.......E. ...

52   In myasthenia gravis

A   there is defective release of acetylcholine at the neuromuscular end-plate

B   there is excessive cholinesterase activity

C   tendon reflexes are normal

D   large doses of neostigmine may cause paralysis

E   thymectomy is more likely to be effective in presence of an adenoma of the thymus

Your answers: A.. ...B.. ..C.. ..D... ..E.: ..

53 **The following are causes of intracranial calcification:**

A   haemangioma
B   hypothyroidism
C   congenital toxoplasmosis
D   pituitary adenoma
E   tuberculoma

Your answers: A.... ..B.. ..C.. ..D......E.. ..

54 **Ulcerative colitis is classically characterised by**

A   fistula formation
B   diarrhoea
C   cobblestoning of mucosa
D   pseudopolyps
E   rectal involvement

Your answers: A.... ..B.. ...C... ..D.. ..E. ...

55 **A male of 60 presents with fatigue, weight loss and serum sodium 120mEq/l. A diagnosis of inappropriate A D H secretion is made. This would be supported by**

A   SG urine never above 1002
B   nocturia
C   serum K 6mEq/l
D   collapse of upper lobe of lung on X-ray
E   B.P. 80/50

Your answers: A.. ..B. ..C.. ...D.. ..E. ...

56 **Circulation of blood through the brain**

A   is uniform throughout the tissue
B   is independent of intracranial pressure
C   is on average 100ml/100g/min in adults
D   is increased by a fall in the pH of extracellular fluid
E   is affected by marked gravitational changes

Your answers: A.... .B... .C......D. ..E.. .

57 **Recognized causes of erythema multiforme include**

A   allergy to drugs
B   viral infection
C   *Mycoplasma pneumoniae*
D   ulcerative colitis
E   acute rheumatic fever

Your answers: A.. ..B.: ..C.. ....D.... .E.......

58 **In the treatment of diabetes mellitus**

A   phenformin is the drug of choice for maturity onset diabetes
B   insulin is never required for maturity onset diabetes
C   coma may be precipitated by glibenclamide
D   chlorpropamide can cause jaundice
E   large doses of insulin are required in hyperosmolar coma

Your answers: A... .B... .C......D.. ...E.. .

59 **Gastrin**

A   is produced in the gastric antrum, jejunum and pancreatic islets in the normal adult
B   is released from the gastric antrum by the stimulus of a falling intra-gastric pH.
C   acts directly on parietal cells and its effect is not reduced by H_2 receptor antagonists (e.g. cimetidine)
D   serum gastrin level is raised in chronic renal failure
E   fasting serum level is higher in patients with pernicious anaemia than in patients with duodenal ulcer

Your answers: A... ..B.......C.......D.......E.. ...

60 **The following statements are correct:**

A   atenolol is at least as selective as practolol as an antagonist at cardiac rather than bronchial and vascular adrenoceptors

B   ipratropium is at least as effective as salbutamol in patients with airways obstruction in chronic bronchitis

C   oral sustained release theophylline is at least as effective as aminophylline suppositories in preventing early morning wheezing

D   orciprenaline is at least as selective as salbutamol for bronchial smooth muscle rather than heart muscle

E   slow intravenous infusion of corticosteroid is at least as effective as the same dose given by intravenous injection in the management of status asthmaticus

Your answers: A.   ...B..   ..C.,   ...D...   ...E.

END OF EXAM 4

Go over your answers until your time is up. Answers and Explanations are on page 110.

PRACTICE EXAM 5

Time allowed 2½ hours.

1 Sacro-iliac joints are liable to be involved in

A ulcerative colitis
B ankylosing spondilitis
C Reiter's syndrome
D sarcoidosis
E psoriasis

Your answers: A.. T.B.. T.C ... ...D. F .E. F...

2 Glycosuria in the elderly

A may result in vulvovaginitis
B usually needs treatment with insulin
C is common because of the lower renal threshold
D is usually associated with ketosis
E indicates diabetes if a single blood glucose determination at the same time is above 10 mmol/1

Your answers: A.... T ..B.. F. C... – D... F...E... F.

3 Regarding cranial diabetes insipidus

A destruction of the posterior lobe of the pituitary results in the diabetes insipidus being permanent
B symptoms may be masked by destruction of the anterior lobe of the pituitary
C cranial diabetes insipidus may be due to lithium toxicity
D the usual treatment is intramuscular injection of synthetic DDAVP (des-amino, d-arginine, vasopressin)
E patients with cranial diabetes insipidus who are deprived access to fluids are at risk of severe hypertonic dehydration

Your answers: A.. F.B.... T.C.. F.D... -.E. T..

4 Achondroplasia

A affects the whole of the skull
B does not reduce sitting height
C inheritance is autosomal recessive
D causes spontaneous fractures
E causes muscle weakness

Your answers: A.... F.B... T. C.. F.D.. F.E. F.

5   Herpetiform enanthem occurs in the following:

A   herpes zoster
B   herpes simplex
C   herpangina
D   measles
E   dermatitis herpetiformis

Your answers: A.......B... ...C.. ..D.......E.......

6   Syringomyelia causes

A   loss of proprioception
B   wasting of small muscles of hands
C   Horner's syndrome
D   loss of reflexes in the upper limbs
E   extensor plantar response

Your answers: A.... ..B.. T.C.......D.. T.E... .

7   In acute myocardial infarction (AMI)

A   coronary care units (CCU's) have had only a slight effect on overall mortality
B   anticoagulation is of little benefit
C   when complete heart block complicates an anterior myocardial infarct the outcome is helped by a pacemaker
D   hypovolaemia may be responsible for hypotension
E   diabetics are not at particular risk after the first week

Your answers: A.......B... F.C...T.D.. T.E.. F.

8   Precipitating antibodies are present in

A   byssinosis
B   bagassosis
C   histoplasmosis
D   fibrosing alveolitis
E   bird fancier's lung

Your answers: A...T...B..: .C.. D. F .E.T ..

9 **Marrow trephine biopsy is more satisfactory than marrow aspiration in the diagnosis of**

    A   aplastic anaemia
    B   sideroblastic anaemia
    C   macrocytic anaemia
    D   marrow involvement in Hodgkin's disease
    E   myelosclerosis

Your answers: A... ..B.. ...C... ...D.. ..E.....

10 **The carpal tunnel syndrome (compression of the median nerve by the flexor retinaculum) will usually cause**

    A   wasting of adductor pollicis
    B   wasting of opponens pollicis
    C   wasting of flexor pollicis longus
    D   sensory loss over the skin of the ring finger
    E   sensory loss over the thenar eminence

Your answers: A.. ...B.. ..C......D... ..E.. ...

11 **Drug induced tardive dyskinesia**

    A   is a long term consequence of blockade of central dopamine receptors
    B   is commonly attributable to antipsychotic drugs of both the butyrophenone and phenothiazine group
    C   can be briefly suppressed by single doses of metoclopramide
    D   can be briefly suppressed by single doses of atropine-like drugs
    E   rapidly resolves after discontinuation of the responsible drug

Your answers: A. ..B. ...C... ..D. ...E.. ..

12 **Calcaneal spurs are a recognised finding in**

    A   tertiary syphilis
    B   Reiter's syndrome
    C   fractures of the calcaneum
    D   Paget's disease
    E   ankylosing spondylitis

Your answers: A... ...B..: ..C... .D... ..E.. ..

13 **T$_3$ (tri-iodothyronine)**

A   is predominantly produced from T$_4$ (thyroxine) in the periphery
B   toxicosis is associated with a normal TSH response to thyrotrophin releasing hormone (TRH)
C   serum levels may be normal in hypothyroidism
D   toxicosis is a commoner form of thyrotoxicosis in iodine deficient areas than in non-iodine deficient areas
E   has a longer biological half life than T$_4$

Your answers: A.. ...B... ...C... .D... ..E.......

14   **The following conditions predispose to the development of osteoarthrosis:**

A   Paget's disease of the bone
B   acromegaly
C   Ehlers - Danlos syndrome
D   aseptic necrosis of the femoral head
E   ingestion of the rye fungus, *Fusarium sparotrichiella*

Your answers: A...'......ß.. ...C... ...D.. ....E.......

15   **A 66 year old lady presents with oedema. The following biochemical abnormalities are noted:- Serum sodium 118 mmol/1. Serum potassium 8.0 mmol/1. Blood urea 7.0 mmol/1. Serum albumin 18 g/1. Serum globulin 20g/1.**

A   hypotraemia is due to inappropriate ADH secretion
B   hyperkalaemia could be iatrogenic in origin
C   an abnormality on chest X-ray would be expected
D   urine testing may be helpful in diagnosis
E   the treatment required is immediate water restriction

Your answers: A. ...B.: ..C. ...D.: .E...

16   **In measles**

A   the rash typically follows three to five days after the prodromal symptoms
B   Koplik's spots are characteristically petechial
C   deaths are usually due to secondary bacterial infection
D   giant cell pneumonia is a recognised complication
E   a blood lymphocytosis is a characteristic finding

Your answers: A.......B.....» C. .D.... E..:

17 Korsakoff's psychosis

A is always a chronic condition
B may be caused by head injury
C is associated with clouding of consciousness
D is characterised by confabulation
E shows gross impairment of intellectual capacity

Your answers: A.......B.....C.   ..D.. ..E..   ..

18 Children may complain of chest pain in the following conditions:

A asthma
B pericarditis
C epidemic pleurodynia
D shingles
E Fallot's tetralogy

Your answers: A.....B.....C.. ..D ....E. .

19 Myotonia

A may occur in Duchenne muscular dystrophy
B may occur in hyperkalaemic periodic paralysis
C may occur in McArdle's disease
D may be treated with procainamide
E may cause no symptoms

Your answers: A.   ..B.. ..C..   D   E..   ..

20 Sino-atrial disease (the sick sinus syndrome) has the following features:

A ventricular dysrhythmias are common
B sinus bradycardia
C high incidence of systemic emboli
D anti-arrhythmic drug treatment is successful
E prognosis is poor

Your answers: A..   ...B.. ..C. ....D... ..E..   .

21 **The following are recognized presenting symptoms of carcinoma of the bronchus without metastases:**

A   tetany
B   painful wrists and ankles
C   ataxia
D   thirst
E   increased skin pigmentation

Your answers: A... B.. C.. ..D.. ...E.. ...

22 **The cause of thrombocytopenia in the following conditions is correctly assigned in each case:**

A   acute leukaemia: marrow aplasia
B   systemic lupus erythematosus: platelet antibodies
C   gram-negative septicaemia: marrow aplasia
D   massive transfusion: platelet antibodies
E   splenomegaly from any cause: sequestration

Your answers: A.. ...B.. ..C.. ..D... .E.: ..

23 **Infections with bacteroides fragilis are amenable to therapy with**

A   metronidazole
B   gentamicin
C   benzyl penicillin
D   clindamycin
E   cephaloridine

Your answers: A.: ...B. ..C. ..D.. ...E... ..

24 **Parkinson-like extrapyramidal effects occur during treatment with**

A   haloperidol
B   imipramine
C   perphenazine
D   phenytoin
E   trifluoperazine

Your answers: A .: .B. ...C.. ...D.. ..E... .

25   A lesion of the common peroneal nerve may

A   be produced by a fracture of the neck of the fibula
B   abolish active extension of the hallux
C   cause foot drop
D   abolish inversion of the foot
E   produce anaesthesia of the sole of the foot

Your answers: A.. ..B.. ..C.. ...D.......E... ..

26   The following statements are true of endogenous depression:

A   it is an illness of rapid onset
B   weight loss is unusual
C   over 90% cases respond to appropriate drug therapy
D   pyschomotor retardation is invariably seen
E   patients have difficulty getting off to sleep

Your answers: A.. ...B.. ...C.. ..D.../ .E.. ...

27   In a teenage patient presenting with short stature

A   raised TSH suggests hypothyroidism
B   Klinefelter's syndrome must be excluded
C   hypogonadism excludes growth hormone deficiency
D   anaemia suggests coeliac disease
E   A 45X karyotype precludes oestrogen treatment until normal
     height is reached

Your answers: A.......B. ....C.. ...D... ..E....

28   Candida albicans infection

A   may give oesophagitis
B   responds to griseofulvin when affecting the nail bed
C   is encouraged by renal glycosuria
D   may produce a nappy rash
E   is responsive to clotrimazole therapy

Your answers: A.... .B.. ..C.. ..D.. ..E....

29   Gout may be associated with

A   polycythaemia rubra vera (PRV)
B   lead poisoning
C   glycogen storage disease (type 1)
D   acromegaly
E   chronic renal failure

Your answers: A. ....B. ....C.. ..D.' ...E.. ...

30   Diffuse oesophageal spasm may be characterised by

A   central chest pain relieved by glyceryl trinitrate
B   effort related pain
C   the presence of a corkscrew oesophagus on barium swallow
D   the absence of simultaneous contractions on manometry
E   a low incidence below the age of 50

Your answers: A. ....B... ..C.. ..D... ..E.... .

31   The following favour a lesion of the brain stem rather than of the cerebral cortex:

A   grasp reflex
B   vertigo
C   diplopia
D   hemiplegia more marked in the arm than in the leg
E   dysarthria

Your answers: A... ...B... ..C.. '' ...E.

32   In myocardial infarction

A   major surgery three months afterwards is followed by reinfarction in 5% of cases
B   90% of myocardial infarcts are recognised clinically at the time
C   vomiting provides an index of the severity of the infarct
D   when the ECG reveals left bundle branch block (LBBB) an infarct can be reliably diagnosed
E   the CK-MM isoenzyme is specific to the myocardium

Your answers: A. ...B.. ..C... ..D.. ...E....

33 Hepatitis B Virus:

A   the surface antigen (HBsAg) is the infective part of the virus
B   the presence of e antigen indicates increased infectivity
C   it is an RNA virus
D   chronic carriers have a risk of developing hepatomas
E   it can be transmitted by insects

Your answers: A.......B.. ...C.. ...D.. ...E.. ..

34 The following statements concerning asbestosis are true:

A   it occurs only in those working in asbestos factories
B   pleural plaques are pre-malignant
C   carcinoma of the bronchus is a recognised complication
D   it is frequently associated with positive antinuclear factor
E   it produces pulmonary nodules as well as marked fibrosis

Your answers: A.. ...B.. ...C.. .D.. ...E.......

35 Pancytopenia may be caused by

A   folic acid deficiency
B   paroxysmal nocturnal haemoglobinuria
C   brucellosis
D   acute myeloblastic leukaemia
E   haemosiderosis

Your answers: A... ...B...   C.......D... ..E.......

36 Parkinson's syndrome may be produced by

A   carbon monoxide poisoning
B   mercury poisoning
C   phenothiazine toxicity
D   vertebro-basilar artery occlusion
E   contraceptive pill

Your answers: A... ...B.. ..C.......D.......E.. ...

37 Endogenous depression will respond to treatment with

A   amitriptyline
B   benztropine
C   electroconvulsive therapy (ECT)
D   flavoxate
E   maprotiline

Your answers: A.......B...   ʳ.. ..D... ..E.......

38 The ureter

A   contains circular and longitudinal smooth muscle arranged in
    spirals
B   is lined with columnar epithelium
C   receives its sympathetic nerve supply from L2, L3 and L4
D   develops from the mesonephric duct
E   radiologically lies on the tips of the transverse processes of the
    lumbar vertebrae

Your answers: A.:.....B..' ..C......D..: ......

39 A high plasma inorganic phosphate level is found in

A   acromegaly
B   renal failure
C   hypoparathyroidism
D   rickets
E   Paget's disease

Your answers: A.......B.. ..C.:. ..D..: ..E.{...

40 Conditions associated with autoimmune thyroid disease include

A   vitiligo
B   alopecia areata
C   premature ovarian failure
D   Turner's syndrome
E   Addisonian pernicious anaemia

Your answers: A.......B.. ..C.: ..D.. ..E. ...

41   Nail changes are a recognised feature of

A   nephrotic syndrome
B   psoriasis
C   subacute bacterial endocarditis
D   alopecia areata
E   pityriasis versicolor

Your answers: A.......B.. ..C.. ..D... F.......

42   Carbon dioxide carriage in the blood is

A   principally in simple solution
B   more than 60% as bicarbonate
C   as carbamino compounds in red cells only
D   dependent on the oxygen saturation of haemoglobin
E   unaffected in early fibrosing alveolitis

Your answers: A.......B......C.. ..D... ..E. ..

43   The following are complications of renal transplantation:

A   necrosis of the femoral head
B   hirsutes
C   visual impairment due to macular degeneration
D   retardation of growth
E   squamous cell carcinoma of the skin

Your answers: A... ...B... ..C.......D.. ..F ..

44   Causes of rectal bleeding in children include

A   polyposis coli
B   constipation
C   intussusception
D   haemophilia
E   Meckel's diverticulum

Your answers: A... ...B... .C.. ..D... ...E. ...

45 In Charcot-Marie Tooth disease

A   clinical manifestations usually first appear in the 4th decade
B   the usual mode of inheritance is autosomal dominant
C   clinical signs appear first in the legs
D   the interossei muscles in the hands are spared
E   progression is slow over many years

Your answers: A.......B.......C. ...D.......E.......

46 Characteristic features of hypertrophic obstructive cardiomyopathy (HOCM) include

A   bisferiens carotid pulse
B   systolic murmur at lower left sternal edge
C   loud fourth heart sound
D   Q waves in the ECG
E   postural syncope

Your answers: A.......B... C.... D.......E.. ...

47 In extrinsic allergic alveolitis

A   there may be sputum eosinophilia
B   type IV hypersensitivity is involved
C   there may be asymptomatic pulmonary insufficiency for several years
D   rheumatoid factor is positive in 30%
E   systemic symptoms typically occur within 20 minutes of exposure to organic dusts

Your answers: A.......B... C... .D... ...E. ...

48 In severe paracetamol poisoning

A   the hepatotoxin is a metabolite rather than paracetamol itself
B   plasma paracetamol concentrations give a useful guide to prognosis
C   the earliest evidence of liver damage is a rise in plasma transaminase concentration
D   acetylcysteine is effective only if given intravenously
E   hepatic coma responds to treatment with neomycin and lactulose

Your answers: A... ..B... ..C... ..D... .E.. ..

49 **In the treatment of chronic granulocytic leukaemia**

A the drug of choice is busulphan
B radiotherapy may be useful in the later stages
C splenectomy is never indicated
D corticosteroids are effective in reducing the cell mass
E fatal marrow hypoplasia is a recognized complication

Your answers: A.....B.....C.....D.....E.....

50 **In sleep disturbance the following statements are valid:**

A 50% of insomnias are secondary
B alcohol increases total sleep time
C benzodiazepine may cause tardive dyskinesia
D narcolepsy usually presents in the lst - 2nd decade
E patients with hypersomnia have an irresistible urge to sleep

Your answers: A.....B.....C.....D.....E.....

51 **Pain and redness are prominent symptoms in the following conditions:**

A conjunctivitis
B acute glaucoma
C subconjunctival haemorrhage
D iritis
E trigeminal neuralgia

Your answers: A.....B.....C.....D.....E.....

52 **Oxygen debt**

A may be 6 times the basal oxygen consumption
B in trained athletes is greater than in an untrained person for a given amount of exertion
C is limited by an increase in pH
D is incurred because blood cannot be delivered to the muscle at a fast enough rate
E is possible because muscle is capable of anaerobic metabolism

Your answers: A.....B.....C.....D.....E.....

53 **The following statements are true of renal tubular disorders:**

A cystine stones and pure uric acid stones cannot be seen on a plain abdominal radiograph
B glycosuria is a common accompaniment of cystinuria
C hypokalaemia is a common accompaniment of renal tubular acidosis
D renal cortical adenyl cyclase deficiency is twice as common in females as males
E treatment of cystinuria may be hampered by the development of proteinuria

Your answers: A.......B... C.......D.......E........

54 **The following are true of autoimmune liver disease:**

A it is more common in females
B chronic active hepatitis occurs in an older age group than primary biliary cirrhosis
C primary biliary cirrhosis responds well to steroids
D an antimitochondrial antibody excludes the diagnosis of chronic active hepatitis
E DNA binding may be increased in both primary biliary cirrhosis and chronic active hepatitis

Your answers: A.. ....B... ..C... ..D... ..E... ..

55 **In the United Kingdom the following immunizations are routinely recommended for children:**

A whooping cough
B tetanus
C BCG
D TAB
E rubella

Your answers: A... ..B... .C... .D.. ...E... ..

56 **Paralysis of the left 3rd cranial nerve causes**

A constricted pupil on the left
B ptosis on the left
C normal direct light reflex on the left
D absence of sweating on the left side of the face
E inability to abduct the left eye

Your answers: A.... ..B.. ..C.. ..D... .E.. ..

57   In patients with sarcoidosis

A   erythema nodosum correlates with a positive Kveim test
B   unilateral hilar adenopathy is a frequent presentation
C   diffuse pulmonary involvement without any symptoms is common
D   heart failure is usually due to primary myocardial involvement
E   bone involvement is associated with hypercalcaemia

Your answers: A.......B.   ..C.: ....D.......E..˙ ...

58   The following statements are true of diazepam:

A   tolerance develops to its actions
B   it can cause physical dependence (addiction)
C   it can induce liver microsomal enzymes
D   it can depress the medulla oblongata
E   it is the drug of choice in status epilepticus

Your answers: A.:.....B..: .C.(..D.(..)E.. ...

59   Which of the following statements are correct:

A   the inter-quartile range contains 95% of the data
B   a confidence interval is the difference between the mean and the median
C   If $p = 0.1$ in a two-tailed test the result is statistically significant
D   a scatterdiagram is for displaying bivariate data
E   a coefficient of variation of 100% implies accurate precision

Your answers: A.......B.......C.......   ......E.......

60   A plasma bicarbonate level of 32 mEq/1

A   is consistent with a diagnosis of chronic cor pulmonale
B   and a serum potassium of 2.7 mEq/1 is consistent with a urine pH of 5.6
C   is a common finding in 21 hydroxylase deficiency
D   is an expected finding in a patient with a ureteric transplant into the sigmoid colon
E   may be associated with tetany

Your answers: A...˙ .B... ..C..( )D.......E..:...

END OF EXAM 5

Go over your answers until your time is up. Answers and Explanations are on page 121.

ANSWERS AND EXPLANATIONS

PRACTICE EXAM I

The correct answer options are given against each question.

1 **B C D E**
If the disease is symptomless bacteria are usually confined to the Ghon focus and will not be found in bronchial (or gastric) secretions. Chemotherapy will tend to prevent complications and the formation of a chronic infective nidus.

2 **A B C**
Exophthalmos may be bilateral or unilateral and the commonest cause is Grave's disease. When due to Grave's disease it may be associated with the hypothyroid, euthyroid or thyrotoxic state. Exposure keratitis may occur when lid apposition is prevented due to exophthalmos and often lid retraction. Various methods of treatment have been advocated including high dose steroids, surgical decompression of the orbit and retro-orbital irradiation, but no method is universally successful. Exophthalmos due to Grave's disease does not vary spontaneously and is often remarkably persistent.

3 **B D**
The fundamental features of acute nephritis include haematuria, oliguria and salt and water retention with resultant oedema and a raised jugular venous pressure. Uraemia in the elderly may lead to diarrhoea and vomiting but despite this, hyperkalaemia is a much more likely accompaniment of oliguria. Complement activation generally results in a lowering of Serum C_3 and CH50 which is restored to normal within 3 months. Persistent reduction of Serum C_3 complement is characteristic of mesangio-capillary (membrano proliferative) nephritis which is more common in the younger population.

4 **A B C D E**
Hypercalcaemia may occur in patients with extensive Paget's disease when immobilized. Deafness may be due either to direct pagetic involvement of the ossicles of the inner ear or to pressure on the eighth cranial nerve by pagetic bone. Overgrowth of pagetic bone at the base of the skull may lead to brainstem compression. Angioid streaks in the retina are found very rarely in Paget's disease and much more often in pseudoxanthoma elasticum. Radiologically both lytic and sclerotic phases are recognized: the lytic phase may be well defined in the calvarium of the skull and then is called osteoporosis circumscripta.

5 C D E

The characteristic ocular abnormality in Wilson's disease is the Kayser-Fleischer ring due to copper accumulation in the cornea. As the disease progresses liver damage occurs and the pathological changes of chronic active hepatitis or postnecrotic cirrhosis become evident. Osteomalacia, sub-articular cysts and fragmentation of the bone in small joints may occur. Biochemically there is a reduced plasma caeruloplasmin and an increased urinary excretion of copper.

6 B E

The aortic arch develops from the fourth left pharyngeal arch, the third becomes the internal carotid. In the fetus, the arch and the pulmonary artery are in communication via the ductus arteriosus which normally shrivels into the fibrous ligamentum arteriosum of the adult. The arch of the aorta is by definition only in the superior mediastinum; it is the descending aorta which lies in the posterior mediastinum below T4 vertebral level.

7 A C

The incidence of hepatitis with Isoniazid in standard first line therapy is only 2% and is acceptable in view of the undoubted benefit. Rifampicin colours the urine, sweat and sputum red and may lead to failure of oral contraception and patients should be warned of these problems. Renal failure may lead to dangerously high levels of Ethambutol. PAS in the urine colours phenistix reddish-purple.

8 C D

Duchenne muscular dystrophy is inherited as an X-linked recesssive and symptoms usually manifest before the age of 5 years. Proximal muscles are affected early, giving difficulty in rising, a waddling gait and frequent falls. The creatinine phosphokinase levels are very high. Myotonia is not a feature. Pseudohypertrophy of the calf muscles is often a very early physical sign in which the affected muscles are enlarged although weak.

9 A B C D

A posterior inferior cerebellar artery thrombosis causes infarction of the nucleus ambiguus and paralysis of the semi-abducted vocal fold. This makes normal speech difficult. Damage to the uncrossed spinal tract of V gives ipsilateral loss of pain and temperature whereas the loss on the opposite side of the body is due to damage to the crossed spinal lemniscus. A palatal palsy is due to bulbar palsy. Vision is not affected as the tracts and nuclei involved in movements of the eyeball lie cephalad in the midbrain and upper pons.

10 A E
Anorexia nervosa classically occurs in post-pubertal girls and is twenty times less common in males. Excessive growth of fine lanugo hair occurs and skin purpura secondary to minor trauma may occur.

11 A B E
Osteoporosis and osteomalacia are common problems in old age and lead to an increased risk of fracture. Osteopetrosis is rarely seen in old age. Osteitis deformans (Paget's disease) is increasingly common with advancing age and is associated with increased numbers of fractures which are often partial.

12 A B C E
Menorrhagia and normochromic anaemia are not uncommon complications of hypothyroidism. Macrocytosis and iron-deficiency anaemia are also well-recognized complications. Clinically significant ascites and cerebellar ataxia are rare. Clubbing and pretibial myxoedema are rare complications of thyrotoxicosis and, if seen, occur in conjunction with exophthalmos in thyroid acropachy.

13 B D E
Well circumscribed, painless, superficial reddened erosions occur on the penis, usually on the glans (circinate balanitis) but sometimes more extensively. Conjunctivitis is the more characteristic eye lesion, but anterior uveitis and (rarely) superficial keratitis may also occur. Subungual keratosis is usually associated with keratodermia blennorrhagica affecting the soles and sometimes the palms.

14 B C E
Parents who batter their children are usually not suffering from a psychotic illness. They often come from unhappy homes and may themselves have been battered as children. Abused children tend to be very young and many show other signs of emotional or physical neglect.

15 B D E
Myasthenia gravis is characterised by abnormal fatiguability of muscles. The predilection is for ocular muscles and others of cranial nerve innervation. Ptosis, strabismus, double vision, dysarthria and dysphagia are common. The symptoms tend to fluctuate, the weakness being aggravated by repeated use of the muscle.
Muscular wasting and sensory deficits are not seen in myasthenia gravis.

16 A B C D

An apical lung tumour can invade the ipsilateral sympathetic fibres (Horner's syndrome), eighth cervical and first thoracic ventral rami (pain in fourth and fifth digits; paralysis of forearm and hand muscles) and the first rib..

17 A B D

All of these cause jaundice of one type or another. Contraceptive steroids probably affect the genetically predisposed. Other formulations of erythromycin seem to be innocent. With methyldopa, jaundice is most commonly hepatocellular and rarely haemolytic.

Prochlorperazine shares the adverse effect associated with chlorpromazine and other phenothiazines. Tetracycline has caused jaundice and fatty liver but chiefly after large parenteral doses in late pregnancy.

18 A C D E

A growth hormone secreting adenoma in the pituitary is the commonest cause of acromegaly. Gonadotrophin deficiency may occur as a result of pituitary destruction, but impotence may be due to hyperprolactinaemia which may also cause galactorrhoea.

Hypercalcaemia and hyperphosphataemia may occur. Cardiomegaly is common in acromegalics due to associated hypertension, higher cardiac output (to keep pace with higher O_2 consumption) or due to cardiomyopathy.

19 B C E

The carcinoid syndrome of cutaneous flushing, diarrhoea, cardiovascular lesions and bronchoconstriction is associated with a tumour, usually of the ileum. Blood pressure may fall during an attack because of the vasodilators (e.g. bradykinin) released. Bronchial carcinoid tumours produce left-sided valve lesions, and more severe flushing. Dietary tryptophan is consumed by the tumour for production of serotonin and thus nicotinamide deficiency can develop leading to pellagra-like skin lesions. It is not unusual for patients to survive for 10 - 15 years after the initial diagnosis.

20 A B E

The onset is abrupt with severe muscle aches. The most prominent signs in the initial leptospiraemic phase of the illness are conjunctival suffusion, neck stiffness, cutaneous haemorrhages and fever; splenomegaly may occur but it is uncommon. Jaundice is common but usually due to a mixture of haemolysis and mild hepatitis.

Death occurs from acute renal failure or haemorrhage. Hepatic failure is not a recognised complication. Organism can be grown in blood cultures although diagnosis is usually made by rising serological titres.

21 B E

Treponema pertenue is the name given to the organism isolated from yaws, although morphologically and antigenically it cannot be distinguished from *Treponema pallidum.* The primary chancre is painless. The secondary stage is characterised by a maculopapular rash, mucous patches, condylomata lata, immune complex glomerulonephritis, arthritis, iridocyclitis, and alopecia. This is the bacteraemic stage when serological tests are almost invariably positive.

22 A D

A radial nerve lesion above the elbow leads to wrist drop and paralysis of the extensor pollicis brevis. Sensory loss is on the dorsum of the hand over the 'anatomical snuff box'. Supination of the flexed forearm is achieved by biceps which is innervated by the musculocutaneous nerve. The interossei are supplied by the ulnar nerve.

23 A C

All are causes of macrocytosis. Tropical sprue produces malabsorption. In pernicious anemia serum folate levels are normal or high. The megaloblastic anemia of pregnancy or alcoholism is usually due to dietary deficiency. Lack of thyroxine, liver disease and chronic lung disease can produce macrocytosis with a normal B_{12} and folate level.

24 A C

Hyoscine and the anticholinergic antihistamines are effective in the management of motion sickness and other labyrinthine disorders. Antihistamines and phenothiazines are effective in controlling nausea of pregnancy, whilst the phenothiazines are the drugs of choice in nausea due to radiation and drugs.

25 A B C D E

The most important causes of papilloedema are raised intracranial pressure, inflammation of the optic disc (as in optic neuritis), and malignant hypertension. It also occurs in many other conditions including malignant thyrotoxic eye disease, chronic bronchitis and the Guillain-Barre syndrome. In benign intracranial hypertension, papilloedema is constant, CSF pressure is raised but there are rarely any focal neurological signs. Early papilloedema causes enlargement of the blind spot. Later, concentric visual field loss occurs.
Fluorescein angiography is useful in confirming the diagnosis in difficult cases.

26   A C
Insulin consists of an A-chain of 21 amino acids and a B-chain of 30 amino acids. Human proinsulin is a single chain polypeptide containing 86 amino acids. Proinsulin is broken down by proteolysis with the formation of insulin and C-peptide. There is an inverse relationship between the growth hormone and blood glucose level, therefore insulin-induced hypoglycaemia causes a rise in growth hormone levels. The sulphonylureas primarily act by stimulating any residual capacity of the cells of the islets to produce insulin.

27   B D
Crohn's disease is favoured by the clinical findings of normal or patchy mucosal changes on sigmoidoscopy and perianal disease.
Biopsy often reveals granulomata in Crohn's disease and crypt abscesses in ulcerative colitis. Radiology showing discontinuous colonic involvement or small bowel involvement would suggest Crohn's.
Toxic dilatation of the colon occurs in both diseases but is rarer in Crohn's disease.

28   A B C
The hypogammaglobulinaemia is due to the arrested stage of development of the 'B' type lymphoid cell in C L L which gives rise to occasional development of autoimmune antibodies. Blast cell transformation is the usual termination in C M L and in 20% of cases is of lymphoblastic type.

29   A B D
Xanthomas occur in the tendons, particularly Achilles, and plantar, patellar and digital extensors of the hands. Early onset of corneal arcus is common. The homozygous state may be complicated by calcific aortic stenosis. Pancreatitis may occur in mixed hypertriglyceridaemia (type V) or in familial lipoprotein lipase deficiency (type I). The serum may be opalescent in Broad-Beta disease (type III), familial lipoprotein lipase deficiency (type I), and endogenous (type IV) and mixed hypertriglyceridaemia (type V).

30   A C D
Chlamydia have a discrete cell wall, contain DNA and RNA and are considered bacterial, despite being obligatory intracellular parasites due to inability to synthesize ATP.
Most are sensitive to sulphonamides but the species *Chlamydia psittaci,* which is harboured by birds and causes psittacosis, is not. Approximately 50% of cases of NGU are due to *Chlamydia trachomatis.*
Trichomoniasis is caused by the protozoin *T. vaginalis. Chlamydia trachomatis* species cause trachoma.

31   B E

The afferent light-reflex fibres run via the optic nerve and optic tract to the pretectal nucleus in front of the mid-brain; they leave the main visual pathway before it reaches the lateral geniculate body. Efferent fibres are from the oculomotor nuclei.

32   B C

In left ventricular failure interstitial pulmonary oedema interferes with gas transfer. Alveolar PCO_2 is increased only when the fluid has entered terminal airways. As the left ventricle fails left ventricular end-diastolic pressure and pulmonary venous pressure rise. X-ray changes may antedate auscultatory findings by 24 hours, depending on the rapidity of onset.

33   B D E

The right main bronchus leaves the trachea at the angle closer to the vertical than the left, and therefore the right lung is more commonly affected. Material is often aspirated into the posterior segments of the upper lobes and the apical segments of the lower lobes. The basal segments of the lower lobe are often spared as the patient is usually lying down when aspiration occurs.

34   B E

Haemosiderinuria only occurs in intravascular haemolysis not necessarily in immune type. The folic acid deficiency may be present as in any haemolytic process. This disease is frequently self limiting without specific therapy, e.g. induced by methyldopa. Only about 50% respond to splenectomy. The fragility of red cells is usually increased due to high reticulocyte count.

35   A B E

Salicylate induced coma is usually a terminal event. Diuresis has no effect on the plasma concentration half time of benzodiazepine. Pentazocine has both agonist and antagonist properties but can nevertheless cause respiratory depression; naloxone is a pure antagonist. The membrane stabilising effects of phenytoin can terminate digoxin induced tachyarrhythmias.

36   B

Statistical significance and clinical significance or biological significance are not the same thing. Data that is not statistically significant may be missing a clinically important result e.g. because of insufficient sample size. The doctor may know the date of birth and be influenced whether to enter the patient into that trial. In a single-blind trial it is the assessor who does not know the treatment. There is never any justification for not randomising patients when comparing different treatments in a clinical trial. It is however equally important that the correct sample size be chosen.

Randomising patients to different treatments does not guarantee similar characteristics. Randomising will usually give similar groups but it is always wise to check all base line measurements carefully for compatibility and to take any differences into account in the analysis.

37   A B D

10 -15% of coeliacs have a family history. Coeliac disease may present with a single deficiency such as iron deficiency rather than the fullblown coeliac syndrome. Hyposplenism is a complication leading to the formation of Howell-Jolly bodies. Bile salt deconjugation is very unusual.

38   A B C D E

Opiate analgesics possessing some antagonistic activity are likely to cause dysphoria and unpleasant hallucinations. They will also precipitate the withdrawal syndrome in patients dependent on opiates. They do have a lower dependence liability than opiate analgesics of low efficacy that lack antagonistic activity.

39   A B D E

The essential features of Fallot's tetralogy are pulmonic stenosis with a ventricular septal defect and right-to-left shunt. Pulmonary oligaemia is characteristic. The systolic murmur originates from right ventricular outflow tract obstruction. This is labile and accounts for the syncopal attacks and aggravation of cyanosis by exertion. Squatting relieves dyspnoea; the physiological mechanisms involved are not understood.

40   D E

Seborrhoeic warts may occur in any area where there are pilosebaceous follicles but are seen predominantly on the face or trunk and may be solitary. They undergo malignant change rarely, but an eruption of warts may be precipitated by an inflammatory dermatosis or by internal malignancy. They are non-infective.

41   C D E

Turner's syndrome usually results from nondysjunction of the sex chromosomes. The karyotype has a normal autosomal complement but only one X chromosome. No Barr bodies are therefore seen on buccal smear. The features of Turner's syndrome include primary hypogonadism (due to absent or 'streaky' ovarian tissue), growth retardation, webbing of neck, wide carrying angle and high urinary gonadotrophins. Cyclical oestrogen replacement therapy induces maturation of the external genitalia and promotes uterine bleeding.

42   **B C D E**
Herpes simplex encephalitis prognosis is universally poor.
Chickenpox encephalitis is cerebellar. Herpes simplex often presents
with a fit and the temporal lobe is most often involved. Unilateral total
nerve deafness can follow mumps encephalitis and is the only
reported long term problem.

43   **B E**
Rose spots can appear everywhere but classically occur over the
upper abdomen and lower thorax. They usually appear around the
10th-11th day of the illness and last 3-4 days and are not petechial.

44   **A B C D E**

45   **D E**
Urobilinogen is present in the urine of normal subjects. An excess of
urobilinogen can be detected by Ehrlich aldehyde reagent. An
increase of urobilinogen in the urine occurs in hepato-cellular
dysfunction; urobilinogen disappears from the urine in intrahepatic
obstruction. Urobilinuria is also found with the increased bilirubin
formation of haemolysis. Mild haemolysis is a feature of pernicious
anaemia.

46   **B C E**
Pseudo-gout is the acute and/or chronic synovitis associated with
calcium pyrophosphate dihydrate (CPPD) crystals in the joint fluid.
The CPPD crystals exhibit weak positive birefringence under polarized
light (cf. strong negative birefringence with sodium urate crystals).
Chondrocalcinosis is associated with but distinct from pseudo-gout. It
occurs predominantly in middle aged and elderly women. The knees
are most commonly affected but often other joints including the
intervertebral disc joints may be involved. Usually the cause is
unknown but there are recognized associations with hyperparathyroidism,
haemochromatosis, diabetes mellitus, acromegaly, Wilson's disease
and alkaptonuria.

47   **E**
Using a conventional formula, the corrected serum calcium = 3.3 +
0.02 (40 - 48) = 3.14 mmol/l. which is raised. In sarcoidosis,
hypercalcaemia is due to excess sensitivity to vitamin D and the
parathormone levels are suppressed. Thiazide diuretics reduce urinary
excretion of calcium. In the presence of hypercalcaemia, urinary
calcium will be increased unless there is significant reduction in
glomerular filtration rate. Hyperparathyroidism is associated with a
low serum phosphate.

48   A B D
Lung compliance is a static measure of lung and chest recoil and is expressed as a change in lung volume per unit change in airway pressure. Since it is a static measure, it cannot be determined by using a peak flow meter. It is decreased by pulmonary congestion and increased by emphysema. It is approximately half of normal in a person with one lung, as the lung volume is approximately half.

49   A C D E
Pancreatitic insufficiency in chronic pancreatitis leads to maldigestion of fats and steatorrhoea. Impairment of vitamin D absorption can lead to osteomalacia. 10% of patients have frank diabetes but impairment of glucose tolerance is found in more cases.
Pseudocysts which usually form three to four weeks after an attack of acute pancreatitis are an occasional complication of chronic pancreatitis.

50   A B C E
Perinatal anoxia or trauma produces hippocampal damage which is thought to be an important factor in the development of late temporal lobe epilepsy. The aura to the seizure is frequently complex involving the higher intellectual functions for example deja vu experiences. 3 per second spike and wave pattern on the EEG is characteristic of petit mal.

51   B C
In constrictive pericarditis the patient is characteristically breathless on exertion but not at rest; orthopnoea is slight or absent. Ascites is much more prominent than peripheral oedema. The jugular venous pulse typically rises on inspiration (Kussmaul's sign) and there is a sharp and marked y descent in early diastole, coinciding with the third heart sound or pericardial knock. In long-standing cases of constrictive pericarditis from any cause calcification is common.

52   A C D E
Asbestosis can cause calcified pleural plaques. Chickenpox causes fine nodular calcification. Silicosis causes 'egg shell' calcification in lymph nodes. Collections of haemosiderin containing macrophages can enlarge and calcify in the lung fields in mitral stenosis. The infiltrates in farmer's lung do not calcify.

53   B D E
Reticulocyte response to bleeding or iron therapy is rarely higher than 5%. Spherocytosis produces crises following infection/stress. Sideroblastosis produces ineffective erythropoiesis with a low reticulocyte count. The anaemia of lead poisoning is not due to haemolysis but impaired haem-synthesis; however red cell survival is

decreased and acute haemolytic anaemia occasionally occurs. Methyldopa produces a 20% incidence of positive Coomb's test but haemolysis in only 1% of these.

54   B C
Negligible evidence supports the numerous claims of differences in the pharmacodynamics of the dozen or so available benzodiazepines. They do however differ in their duration of action. Triazolam, temazepam and oxazepam are short-acting (plasma concentration half time less than 10 hours). The remainder persist in the body for a long time, e.g. diazepam (and its active metabolites) with a half time of up to 3 days in the elderly. The cost difference between the most and least expensive is about 10-fold.

55   A C E
Polymyalgia rheumatica almost always occurs in elderly patients. The main complaint is of widespread muscular pain and sometimes general malaise. Muscle weakness is not normally present although movement may be restricted with pain. The ESR is generally elevated. The electromyogram, serum enzme studies and muscle biopsies are usually normal. The response to steroid therapy is immediate and dramatic

56   A B C D
Hypochondriacal ideas may occur as bizarre delusions in schizophrenia or an nihilistic delusions in depression. Hypochondriacal symptoms of a delusional quality may be a feature of dementia. The anxious hypochondriac may be a phobia for a specific disease, e.g. cancer, whilst in obsessive-compulsive neurosis there is an overwhelming preoccupation with bodily health.

57   B C
IRDS may occur at any gestation. When established it does not respond to corticosteroids, although this therapy may be beneficial to certain infants when previously adminstered to the mother whilst the baby is in utero. Intraventricular haemorrhage is often associated with IRDS.

58   A B C
A third heart sound (protodiastolic gallop) and mural thrombosis are common in congestive cardiomyopathy. Alcoholic cardiomyopathy may respond clinically to thiamine, but withdrawal of alcohol is just as important. Dysrhythmias may be difficult to treat. Beta-blockers must be used *very* cautiously since they can precipitate severe pulmonary oedema and cardiogenic shock. Pericardial effusions do not occur.

59 B C D
Crackles are heard in bronchiectasis, pulmonary oedema, left ventricular failure (associated with severe hypertension, valvular heart disease and massive myocardial infarction) and pulmonary fibrosis as in intrinsic or extrinsic allergic alveolitis and sarcoidosis.

60 A B E
In rheumatic fever, carditis is suggested by the presence of diastolic or long systolic murmurs, by pericarditis and by cardiomegaly (pericardial effusion excluded by echocardiography). A prolonged PR interval is very common in rheumatic fever (80%) and is present equally in those with and without carditis. Sinus arrhythmia is a normal finding.

PRACTICE EXAM 2

1 B C D
A variety of organisms can cause this condition. Clioquinol toxicity has been confined to Japan. Peace corps volunteers in Africa were helped by doxycycline. Many patients with colitis recall diarrhoea on holiday, but the experience is equally common amongst non-paitents.

2 A D
In amyloidosis complicating chronic infection, hepatosplenomegaly, hepatic and renal function impairment and nephrotic syndrome may occur. Right ventricular hypertrophy is a feature of cor pulmonale and also of primary amyloid. Clubbing of the fingers is a feature of bronchiectasis.

3 B C D E
Classically the headache of raised intra cranial pressure occurs first thing in the morning, the patient wakening with it and it wears off as the day progresses. It is made worse by factors which raise intra-cranial pressure, e.g. coughing, stooping, straining at stool. Episodes of transient blindness (visual obscurations) indicate markedly elevated intra-cranial pressure.

4 B D
Cannon waves occur when the right atrium contracts against a closed tricuspid valve and have the same timing as a-waves. They occur in complete heart block when atrial and ventricular contractions coincide but not in second degree heart block. Regular cannon waves can occur when nodal activities of the atria delay their contraction to coincide with that of the ventricles. Large a-waves occur in tricuspid stenosis.

5 A B C D
Lesch-Nyhan syndrome is an X-linked genetic disease in which there is deficiency of hypoxanthine-guanine phosphoribosyl- transferase. There is over-production of urate, gout and neurological damage. The serum uric acid is elevated in myeloproliferative disorders such as polycythaemia rubra vera. Hyperuricaemia is also associated with hyperparathyroidism. The hyperuricaemia of starvation results largely from inhibition of renal tubular urate secretion by the accumulated hydroxybutyrate. Hyperuricaemia may be found in hypothyroidism not thyrotoxicosis.

6 A B C D
Common side effects of Bromocriptine therapy are nausea, vomiting and postural hypotension which usually last for only a short time. In normal subjects it causes a rise in serum growth hormone (GH). It lowers the serum prolactin level in normal subjects and in well over 90% of patients with hyperprolactinaemia. In patients with pituitary-dependent Cushing's syndrome it lowers the plasma ACTH concentration in a few but in the majority of cases the ACTH level is unaffected. Bromocriptine can induce some clinical improvement in some patients with acromegaly.

7 A C
Left ventricular activation is slightly ahead of the right. The fourth heart sound occurs in atrial systole but is only rarely heard in a normal heart. The aortic valve cusps float upwards during ventricular filling. As LVEDP rises, stroke work increases proportionally less until a plateau is reached.

8 B C
Escherichia coli accounts for three-quarters of urinary tract infections in general practice. *Proteus mirabilis* infection is common in hospital practice and points to the possibility of renal tract abnormalities, renal calculi, and previous operative interference. Inadequate bladder emptying due to bladder neck obstruction impairs bacterial elimination, the infection arising from faecal organisms ascending from the perineum. In the absence of urinary tract abnormalities, renal calculi, and analgesic abuse urinary tract infection is rarely associated with renal failure.

9 A B C D E
Local complications of ulcerative colitis include fistula-in-ano colonic perforation, colonic dilatation and carcinoma. Systemic complications include arthritis, uveitis, erythema nodosum, pyoderma gangrenosum and aphthous stomatitis. Amyloidosis is an occasional complication.

10   A B C D
Follow up studies into adult life indicate that the disease is peristent. Most authorities agree that jejunal biopsy is essential.

11   C D E
Myotonic dystrophy is inherited as an autosomal dominant character, and affects males and females. Weakness is initially in hands and feet, but progresses proximally. There is almost always selective weakness of the sternomastoids. Ptosis, facial weakness and dysarthria may be seen. Cataracts, testicular atrophy and baldness are other features. Conduction defects on ECG are common and cardiac arrythmias may occur.

12   A D E
In Reiter's syndrome, ankylosing spondylitis and giant-cell arteritis aortitis may result in aortic regurgitation. Aortitis does not develop in polymyalgia rheumatica. Valvular damage from nonbacterial verrucous endocarditis is a recognized complication of systemic lupus erythematosus and can result in aortic regurgition.

13   A B C D E
Weight loss and fever in P.A. may mimic carcinoma of the stomach. The fever if significant is often due to an occult infection. Severe neurological defects due to B_{12} deficiency will only partially resolve on vitamin B_{12}. (C) is correct as manifested by hyperbilirubinemia and high LDH. Serum folate levels are normal or high due to the methyl folate trap. In (E) circulating megaloblasts may be found with thrombocytopenia and leucopenia, and rarely myelocytes are also present.

14   A B D
Reduced cardiac output and antagonism of circulating adrenaline at vascular β- andrenoceptors sub serving vasodilation combine to reduce peripheral blood flow. Not only does restoration of normal blood glucose take longer but also the symptoms of hypoglycaemia are partially masked. Physiological tremor is enhanced by agonists at β-adrenoceptors. Vivid dreams are common; hallucinations and confusional states also occur. Only practolol, of the group, causes the oculo-mucocutaneous syndrome.

15   B E
Delirium tremens is associated with clouding of consciousness, disorientation, loss of recent memory and visual hallucinations. The peak incidence is 72-96 hours after admission to hospital. Korsakoff's psychosis is a frequent sequel.

16   B C E

The predominant influence on prolactin secretion from the pituitary is inhibition by dopamine and probably other factors. Therefore drugs which influence dopamine metabolism or secretion such as reserpine or methyldopa lead to hyperprolactinaemia. Hypothyroidism but not thyrotoxicosis is complicated by hyperprolactinaemia and may rarely present with galactorrhoea and amenorrhoea. A raised serum prolactin level is quite commonly found in acromegaly.

17   A B D E

Congenital toxoplasmosis may cause a choroidoretinitis the significance of which depends on whether there is macular involvement. Cor pulmonale causes retinal vein congestion and papilloedema. The retinopathy associated with chloroquine therapy is characterised by granular pigmentation of the macula and retinal artery constriction. It is progressive and irreversible and may cause blindness. Aortic arch obstruction causes a reduction in retinal artery blood flow and retinal ischaemia. The fundus is not involved in Marfan's syndrome unless there has been a retinal detachment.

18   A B C E

Klinefelter's syndrome is a variety of male hypogonadism characterised by an extra X chromosome, (giving a total number of 47 chromosomes) and a positive buccal smear. Common clinical associations are abnormal tallness, gynaecomastia and mental retardation. Plasma and urinary levels of gonadotrophins are high - a finding which serves to distinguish this type of hypogonadism from that secondary to hypothalamopituitary dysfuntion.

19   A B C D

In both the sympathetic and the parasympathetic nervous system, acetylcholine is the transmitter substance released from the terminals of the preganglionic fibres. Acetylcholine is also the transmitter at neuro-effector junctions. The postganglionic neurones which innervate sweat glands and those which supply blood vessels in skeletal muscles belong anatomically to the sympathetic nervous system, but release acetylcholine. The postganglionic effects of acetylcholine can be reproduced by muscarine. Pseudocholin-esterase is capable of hydro-lysing acetylocholine, but is found in blood, not at nerve endings.

20   A B

A number of systemic disorders are associated with fibrosing alveolitis including SLE, systemic sclerosis, RA, adult coeliac disease and chronic active hepatitis or cirrhosis. Dermatomyositis is associated with fibrosing alveolitis, but may also complicate carcinoma of the lung which itself may complicate fibrosing alveolitis.

21 A B D E
Rheumatoid factors are auto-antibodies specific for the Fc fragment of IgG. IgM rheumatoid factor is positive in the majority of patients with rheumatoid arthritis and may be positive in a variety of other diseases usually characterized by chronic inflammation with persistent antigenic challenge. However patients with psoriatic arthritis are seronegative.

22 A
Accelerated hypertension due to renal stenosis is cause by secondary hyperaldosteronism. Until significant hypertensive damage occurs in the contralateral kidney renal function, both tubular and glomerular, is maintained even when the blood pressure is lowered by the angio-tension convertase inhibitor, Captopril. Diminished renal blood flow increases sodium and water reabsorption and increased pyelographic concentration may occur in the affected kidney.

23 B C E
Regional enteritis (Crohn's disease) can affect any part of the gastro-intestinal tract, and has a remitting and relapsing course.
Fistula formation is a well known complication and steatorrhoea may occur. X-ray appearances include cobblestoning of the mucosa, and narrowing of segments of the small intestine.

24 B C D E
The predominant haemoglobin is type F in all neonates: the thalassaemic state appears later as the child converts from Hb. F to Hb. A. Widespread marrow hyperplasia results in bony overgrowth.
The prognosis is grave and many children fail to survive into adult life.

25 A C E
In addition to hypertension the other risk factors for stroke are heart disease, diabetes and transient ischaemic attacks. These factors can increase the risk factor from 2 to 12 times. Healthy women under the age of 35 who take oral contraceptives have an increased risk of stroke but not of myocardial infarction.

26 B C D
The first heart sound is characteristically soft; when loud it excludes severe mitral regurgitation. The third heart sound and diastolic murmur (in the absence of any stenosis) reflect rapid diastolic filling of the left ventricle. Left atrial distension in systole may produce a left sternal heave. The second heart sound is usually normal; with severe

regurgitation early aortic valve closure causes wide (but not reversed) splitting of the second sound.

27 A B C E
Cheyne-Stokes respiration (periods of apnoea alternating with a series of breaths of increasing then decreasing amplitude) is usually due to brain stem compression with raised intracranial pressure. It may also occur as a result of metabolic upsets (such as cardiac, respiratory or renal failure) and as a result of CNS depressant drug poisoning. In diabetic ketoacidotic coma, the respirations are deep and sighing (Kussmaul).

28 A B E
Serum iron is usually low in presence of increased iron stores. The iron deficiency in Thalassemia minor is due to faulty globin chain synthesis. Splenomegaly in patients with iron deficiency is rarely found in modern practice. Iron deficiency is rare in men and most often due to blood loss not dietary deficiency. (E) is true hence the term bronze diabetes.

29 A D E
Minoxidil is a prodrug, the active metabolite of which dilates arterioles selectively rather than veins. Inactivation is by further liver metabolism. A compensatory increase in heart rate prompts combination therapy. When an antagonist at β-adrenoceptors is contra-indicated methyldopa can be used to reduce the tachycardia.
Hypertrichosis is troublesome in women; it resolves about 3 months after drug withdrawal. The tachycardia can induce angina but the ECG changes are seldom accompanied by symptoms.

30 A B C E
Depression may precede other symptoms of carcinoma of the pancreas by some months. It may also occur in acute viral illness and in diseases associated with dementia such as Huntingdon's chorea. It may occur as part of the aura in temporal lobe epilepsy.

31 A B C D
Permanent diabetes insipidus is due to hypothalamic or high stalk damage. Craniopharyngioma, histiocytosis X and sarcoidosis much more commonly directly involve the hypothalamus rather than the pituitary gland; therefore diabetes insipidus is a well-recognised complication of these conditions. Destruction of the posterior lobe of the pituitary may lead to transient but not permanent diabetes insipidus. Rarely an untreated pituitary adenoma with a large suprasellar extension may lead to diabetes insipidus.

32   A E
The vertebral artery arises as the first branch of the subclavian artery. The artery ascends through the foramen in the transverse processes of the upper 6 cervical vertebrae, curves behind the lateral mass of the atlas and then enters the cranial cavity through the foramen magnum. The arteries join at the lower border of the pons to form the basilar artery. The posterior inferior cerebellar arteries are branches of the vertebral arteries whereas the anterior inferior cerebellar arteries and the superior cerebellar arteries are branches of the basilar artery.

33   ALL FALSE
Emotional or physical trauma may occasionally precede alopecia areata but there is frequently no trigger factor. It may be more common in those of Mongoloid race. In Down's syndrome the hair may be sparse and fine. Hair loss which is commonly asymptomatic in alopecia areata may occur at any site, although scalp hair is more frequently affected. Most of the follicles retain the ability to form new hair and there is no scarring.

34   C D
Meningo-encephalitis is the commonest complication and pancreatitis is very rare. Oophoritis is a well known complication and like orchitis is nearly always unilateral. Encephalitis can be the only clinical manifestation.

35   B C
In polymyalgia rheumatica the proximal muscles ache, are stiff and in the mornings, may be tender, but are not genuinely weak. The serum CPK, electromyogram (EMG) and muscle biopsy are all normal. Diagnosis is based on the clinical features and usually the ESR is markedly elevated.

36   D E
Membranous nephropathy presents as the nephrotic syndrome and patients are rarely hypertensive. Characteristically electron dense deposits are confined to the subepithelial side of the basement membrane. The prognosis is variable; 25 - 30% of patients remit spontaneously. Previous trials have failed to show any benefit from steroid therapy but isolated cases have responded and further trials are currently in progress using higher doses than previously.
Opinions about this question may change. There is a high incidence of associated neoplasia.

37   A C E
Chronic hypochlorhydria leads to hyperplasia of antral gastrin secreting cells (G-cells) and 75% of patients with pernicious anaemia

have raised fasting serum gastrin. The Zollinger-Ellison syndrome is due to a gastrin secreting tumour usually of the pancreas. In duodenal ulcer, fasting gastrin levels are normal but rise more than normal after a protein meal. Patients with gastric ulcer may have mildly raised gastrin levels. The reason serum gastrin is elevated after small bowel resection is not known.

38   A B C D E
Partial or complete sensorineural deafness occurs in about 20% of patients with bacterial meningitis and is especially associated with meningococcal meningitis. Focal or generalised seizures occur in the acute phase of bacterial meningitis in 20 - 30% of patients and may be due to cerebral involvement, penicillin neurotoxicity or high fever in the infant. Ventriculitis probably occurs in most cases.
Hydrocephalus may develop due to obstruction to the CSF flow within the ventricles (obstructive hydrocephalus) or extraventricularly (communicating hydrocephalus). 10 - 20% of patients who recover from the acute illness have residual neurological damage.

39   A B
Polymorphonuclear leucocytosis in the CSF is associated with pyogenic infections. In tuberculous meningitis a mixed cytosis occurs with a high proportion of polymorphs at first but as the disease progresses the proportion of lymphocytes rises steadily until they represent 90% of the total cell count.

40   A B D E
The side effects of digoxin toxicity are protean and often affect elderly patients who have reduced tolerance to the drug. Gastro- intestinal symptoms are prominent with anorexia, vomiting, abdominal pain, diarrhoea and weight loss. Confusion, delirium and seizures may occur. Visual symptoms include alterations in colour vision and even blindness. A wide variety of ventricular and supraventricular rhythms may occur and can be difficult to treat.

41   A C D
Not all inhaled inorganic dusts cause fibrosis of the lung. It is not a feature of simple coal miners pneumoconiosis, siderosis from pure iron oxide inhalation (e.g. in welding) or stannosis (in tin smelting workers). Silica, tungsten carbide and aluminium are fibrogenic dusts.

42   A B
In the diffuse category only small cell type have a good prognosis. The old but commonly used Rappaport classification overestimates

the incidence of true histiocytic lymphoma, most large cell types being lymphoblastic B or T cell malignancies.

43   A D E

Large doses cause cessation of cortisol production and by increasing neuronal excitability can precipitate generalised seizures and acute psychosis. Lymphoid involution and diminution of the immune response contribute to the suppression of transplant rejection.

44   A B D

Neurofibromas may occur on optic nerves leading to optic atrophy, and on auditory nerves leading to deafness. Phaeochromocytomas are occasionally associated with neurofibromatosis and therefore paroxysmal hypertension may occur. Osteosclerosis tibiae is identical with Paget's disease of bone and is not associated.

45   A D

The expected frequencies shall all be greater than 5. The chi-square statistic can be artificially enlarged if the expected frequencies are too small as they are the divisors in the calculation i.e. SUM (obs - exp) < (obs - exp) / exp. A paired t-test would be used in a before/after study of a single variable assuming the data is normally distributed. Non-parametric tests are used when the data is not normally distributed. The Mann-Whitney U-test is equivalent to the unpaired t-test; the paired t-test is equivalent to the Wilcoxon matched-pairs signed-ranks test.

46   A D

Falciparum malaria (cerebral) is the most virulent of the four types of malaria and splenomegaly is an important clinical sign. Acute renal failure is common. There is no dormant liver stage as in vivax, ovale or malariae and recurrence of fever after one year is rare. Tertial periodicity does occur but is far from characteristic.

47   B C

Hypothermia is a common problem in old age. Chlorpromazine and other tranquillisers have a direct effect on the temperature regulating centre, inhibit shivering and cause peripheral vasodilation, all of which make hypothermia worse. Many complications result from hypothermia and acute pacreatitis is more likely with increasing length of time. Vasodilatory drugs would make matters worse and treatment is by slow warming. Reflexes slow in hypothermia and do not indicate hypothyroidism.

48   A C

Calcification of the basal ganglia, cataracts, tetany, epilepsy and papilloedema may complicate hypoparathyroidism. Biochemical investigations reveal a low plasma calcium, raised plasma phosphate and a low or undetectable parathormone concentration. Macrocytosis and anaemia may complicate hypothyroidism but are not a consequence of hypoparathyroiodism.

49   C

Suicide tends to occur in males of the older age group, in contrast to the majority of drug overdoses which occur in young females. The suicide rate has remained relatively constant in recent years. Self-poisoning accounts for about 60% cases while one third use a more violent method. Peak incidence is in the spring.

50   B D

Complement consists of a series of serum globulins with mainly β electrophoretic mobility present in fresh normal serum. The reaction of IgG antibody with antigen allows the first component of complement C1q to bind to the Fc region of the antibody, activating the classical complement sequence. The critical step in complement activation is cleavage of C_3 which is achieved by both the classical and the alternative routes. Patients with hereditary angio-oedema have deficiency of C1q inhibitor. Complement is necessary for the lysis of cells.

51   B C

Legionella pneumophilia is a gram negative bacillus which causes chest infections varying from mild bronchitis to severe pneumonia. Mortality used to be 20% but is now much less because mild cases are being diagnosed. Renal failure is very rare even in fatal cases. Respiratory failure is the commonest cause of death. Long term lung damage has not been recorded.

52   A E

A rheumatoid granuloma or nodule may occur as a solitary lesion in the lung; more often there are multiple nodules in the lung, these tend to be peripheral. Pleural effusions, usually unilateral, tend to occur in elderly men. They are usually associated with subcutaneous nodules and positive rheumatoid factor and may resolve spontaneously. Iritis is not a feature of adult rheumatoid disease. Keratoconjunctivitis sicca, episcleritis and scleritis are the most important ocular manifestations. Glomerulonephritis does not occur in rheumatoid disease. Amyloidosis may occasionally develop in patients with long-standing disease and can result in renal failure.

53 A C E

Three immunotypes of *Chlamydia trachomatis* cause L G V,L$_2$ being the most common. The primary lesion heals within a few days without scarring followed within a few weeks by multicolour suppurative regional lymphadenopathy. Constitutional symptoms are common including meningoencephalitis. Women and homosexual men may develop haemorrhagic proctocolitis. The most reliable method of diagnosis is isolation of the organism from infected tissue or pus but the L G V complement fixation test is helpful and recently a micro-immunofluorescent test has been developed which is more specific. Occasional isolates are resistant to sulphonamides.

54 B C D E

Accumulation of fluid in the peritoneal cavity may be transudate, as in cirrhosis of the liver, constrictive pericarditis, and Meigs's syndrome. In tuberculous peritonitis and carcinonomatous involvement of the peritoneum, it is an exudate, and characteristically has a high protein content.

55 A D E

Threadworms infest the colon. Iron deficiency is a result of malabsorption. A late complication of abdominal radiotherapy in a small proportion of patients is the formation of an intestinal stricture with consequent stasis and steatorrhoea.

56 A B C D E

The pedunculated left atrial myxoma may fall into the mitral orifice and obstruct blood flow into the left ventricle; thus syncope and acute pulmonary oedema may occur. Less often the findings resemble those produced by combined mitral stenosis and regurgitation or even pure mitral regurgitation. Embolic manifestations are common resulting in stroke, peripheral gangrene etc. There is a raised sedimentation rate and hyperglobulinaemia.

57 A C D E

The pulse in respiratory failure is usually a large volume, bounding pulse. All the other features point to a diagnosis of respiratory failure but must be confirmed by arterial blood gas measurements.

58 B D E

Myeloma is associated with lytic bone lesions and consequently pathological fractures. Renal tubular defects occur as a result of immunoglobulin light chains damaging tubular epithelium. Renal function may also be impaired by amyloid, hypercalcaemia, and uric acid crystals deposition.

59 **B C D E**
Less than 20% is absorbed after oral dosage. Enema adminstration is effective. Prostaglandin synthesis in vitro is suppressed not only by the salicylate metabolite but also by the parent compound. Recognised adverse effects include haemolysis and reversible oligospermia.

60 **B E**
The ulnar nerve is derived from spinal nerves C7, C8 and T.1. It supplies flexor carpi ulnaris and half of flexor digitorum profundus in the forearm and the majority of the intrinsic muscles of the hand including the dorsal interossei and hypothenar eminence. The radial nerve is the termination of the posterior cord of the brachial plexus and innervates the extensor muscles of the upper arm and forearm.

PRACTICE EXAM 3

1 **B C D E**
In erythema multiforme lesions with a central necrotic area are characteristic although in more severe forms erythematous plaques with a central bulla (large blister) and marginal ring of vesicles may be present. The most severe variant Stevens-Johnson syndrome usually presents with bullous lesions. Dermatitis herpetiformis is characterised by itchy vesicles arising on normal or erythematous skin. Bullae on light exposed surfaces are seen in porphyria cutanea tarda. In exfoliative dermatitis the skin becomes reddened and then peels without vesicle formation.

2 **E**
Thyroid cancer and hyperthyroidism rarely co-exist. Thyroid cancer is characteristically a 'cold nodule' on radioisotope scanning of the thyroid gland. The commonest cancer in the young patient is a papillary carcinoma and the anaplastic tumours typically occur in the elderly. Follicular carcinomas particularly metastasise to bone and the papillary type carries a better prognosis than the follicular type.

3 **B C E**
Autosomal dominant inheritance takes place through a non sex chromosome, when the character is said to be dominant if the gene controlling it produces the same effect in the heterozygous and homozygous states. This occurs in arachnodactyly, polyposis coli, and dystrophia myotonica. Haemophilia is inherited by a sex linked

recessive mechanism and cystinuria is thought to be inherited by an autosomal recessive mechanism.

4 B D
Renal papillary necrosis is thought to occur in diabetes mellitus due to a combination of dehydration and infection, characteristically staphylococcal, and results in acute loss of renal function. It may occur in both sickle cell disease and sickle cell trait. Medullary sponge kidney has to be distinguished radiologically from papillary necrosis, particularly that associated with analgesic abuse, by the absence of calyceal deformity. The changes are caused by ectasia of the collecting ducts usually associated with small calculi in the pyramids which need to be differentiated from other causes of nephrocalcinosis. Previously sulphonamide derivatives occasionally caused crystalluria. Nowadays sensitivity vasculitis may rarely occur but neither is associated with papillary necrosis. Acute pancreatitis occasionally causes renal cortical necrosis.

5 A
Diverticular disease can present with very heavy rectal bleeding. Pain is only prominent when it is complicated by diverticulitis. Gastro-colic and vesico-colic but not perianal fistulae are recognised complications. Carcinoma is as common in patients with diverticular disease as the general population. The diverticula follow the course of a nutrient artery with the muscularis of the bowel wall and hence are usually on the mesenteric side.

6 A C D
Classically plaques of demyelination occur in areas close to the ventricular system of the brain and in the midbrain lie in the periaqueductal area frequently producing intranuclear ophthalmoplegia. The optic nerves are a frequent site of demyelination as in retrobulbar neuritis. In the spinal cord the cervical segments are much more frequently affected than the thoracic segments. The plaques lie laterally in the cord thus involving the spinothalamic pathways and sparing the posterior columns.

7 A C E
Infective endocarditis may result in an immune-complex nephritis. Combined benzylpenicillin and gentamicin is the treatment of choice in *Streptococcus faecalis* endocarditis. With brucellosis, endocarditis is a rare complication of a rare disease. Splenomegaly may be absent in the early stages. Invasive procedures such as sigmoidoscopy and cystoscopy result in bacteraemia and increase the risk of endocarditis in susceptible subjects.

8   B E
Pneumocystis infection occurs almost exclusively in immunosuppressed patients but rare outbreaks occur in others. Co-trimoxazole is useful in therapy and in prophylaxis. Demonstration of organisms in specimens obtained directly from the lung is usually required for diagnosis. Simultaneous infection with CMV is commonplace.

9   A B C D E
The worsening pruritus is due to histamine release. Iron deficiency is almost invariable. Gout is due to high cellular turnover. Raised leucocyte alkaline phosphatase could be due to infection or thrombosis. Splenomegaly is the only physical finding of diagnostic significance.

10   C D E
Haemolysis provoked by methyldopa is rare (0-0.2%) and acetylator status has no relevance since elimination is mainly by the kidney.
Isoniazid hepatitis may be related to a metabolite since it is more common in fast acetylators. The remaining adverse effects are dose dependent and are more commonly seen in slow acetylators.

11   A D E
The disease often heralds asthma, of which a family history is common. Respiratory syncytial virus is responsible in most cases. Controlled trials have failed to show benefit from corticosteroids.

12   B D E
The spasticity of a pyramidal lesion is more evident in the flexor muscles of the upper limb and in the extensor muscles of the lower limb. A common cause of foot drop is trauma to the common peroneal nerve as it is subcutaneous lateral to the neck of the fibula.

13   C
Hysteria tends to occur in persons with an insecure personality, who tend to opt out of stressful situations by developing illness. The typical mental attitude of "la belle indifference" is not always found and it tends to be a late feature of established disabling symptoms. Hysterical patients do not usually look physically ill.
Apparent hysterical symptoms developing for the first time in middle age or later should raise a high suspicion of organic disease.

14   B C
Conventional non-steroidal anti-inflammatory agents provide symptomatic benefit but have no essential effect on the activity of the disease. There is good evidence that gold therapy modifies the course of the disease, although whether or not it slows down the rate of bony damage is controversial. Patients who are HLA DRW3 positive have

an increased risk of developing nephrotoxicity (proteinuria) during gold or D-penicillamine treatment. Patients with rheumatoid arthritis are prone to develop septic arthritis, irrespective of steroid treatment.

15   A D E

Plasma protein concentration is maintained in starvation. The osmotic pressure of plasma proteins plays an important role in the exchange of fluid across the capillaries, but is only 25mmHg which represents a small proportion of the total osmotic pressure of plasma. Electophoretic mobility is the basis of separation of plasma proteins. In addition to serving as binding proteins for certain hormones, they contribute to the buffering capacity of the blood.

16   A C E

Polycystic kidneys are always enlarged and often huge. Enlargement often occurs following infiltration with amyloid, lymphoma etc. and often occurs transiently following acute tubular necrosis and in acute glomerulonephritis. In both chronic glomerulonephritis and analgesic nephropathy the kidneys are usually symmetrically reduced in size.

17   A C D

Campylobacter infection is a major cause of diarrhoea in both adults and children. It is characterised by abdominal pain which can lead to inappropriate surgery. Sigmoidoscopy and rectal histology can be identical with ulcerative colitis. If treatment is necessary the drug of choice is Erythromycin.

18   A C D

Delirium tremens may be precipitated by acute infection and following operation or accident, the sudden deprivation of alcohol being the most important factor. The alcoholic cerebellar syndrome consists of ataxia of gait and legs with little or no involvement of the arms and rarely dysarthria and nystagmus. Epilepsy can occur either on withdrawal or severe intoxication. Alcoholic dementia does not differ from other patterns of dementia with impairment of memory and intellectual functioning.

19   A C D

Glyceryl trinitrate relaxes vascular smooth muscle. Vasodilatation of the coronary arteries results in improved blood flow to the normal and ischaemic myocardium. Dilatation of the veins causes pooling of blood peripherally, a reduction in ventricular volume and consequently a reduced myocardial oxygen demand. Systemic arterial dilatation may lower the arterial blood pressure, particularly on standing. Methaemoglobinaemia may occur if large doses are taken.
Glyceryl trinitrate is effective for about 30 minutes when taken sublingually.

20 A B C

Legionella pneumophilia is a small gram negative cocco-bacillus.
Prodromal symptoms often include abdominal pain and diarrhoea. A
lymphopenia may occur with a moderate leucocytosis. Microscopic
haematuria occurs in approximately 50% of patients. Erythromycin
is the treatment of choice.

21 D

In von Willebrand's disease bleeding is due to a qualitative defect of
platelet aggregation due to decreased factor VIII Antigen.
Aspirin decreases thromboxane synthesis even in low doses; it is
rarely reported to produce thrombocytopenia. Goodpasture's syndrome
produces lung haemorrhage and platelet consumption.
Oxyphenylbutazone, like all Pyrazole derivatives may produce
aplasia.
Bleeding in scurvy is usually associated with folate deficiency which
exacerbates the thrombocytopenia.

22 A B D E

The cardiac effects of calcium ion and digitalis are very similar.
Hyperkalaemia promotes A-V block whereas hypokalaemia and
hypomagnesaemia (separately or in combination) favour ectopic
rhythms. Predictably, replacement of potassium deficit diminishes
ectopic activity but does not reduce A-V block. Hypoalbuminaemia
has no direct relevance to the handling of digoxin which is not
extensively bound to plasma protein.

23 A E

The synovial fluid contains predominantly polymorphs - up to 50,000
per mm^3 and consequently appears turbid.
Rheumatoid factors are autoantibodies against the Fc fragment of
IgG. The standard tests detect the presence of IgM rheumatoid
factors. 80% of patients with rheumatoid arthritis are seropositive,
yet only 20% have rheumatoid nodules. Those patients with rheumatoid
nodules or a digital infarct are almost always seropositive. Rheumatoid
arthritis of the knee predisposes to the formation of a Baker's cyst
which can rupture into the calf muscles and mimic a deep vein
thrombosis.

24 A B C E

In *Schistosma haematobium* infection the urinary system is affected
most. Bladder calcification and calculi cause hydronephrosis in up to
30% of chronic cases and renal parenchymal disease also occurs.
Penetration of the larvae through the skin causes internal irritation
and allergic manifestation such as eosinophilia are very common.

Trivalent antimony (not arsenical) compounds used to be used successfully in treatment.

25   **C D**
Arterioslerotic dementia differs from senile dementia in its relatively acute onset and stepwise progression. It tends to affect a younger group of patients than senile dementia. The condition is patchy and insight is often retained. Depression and emotional lability are common accompaniments.

26   **NONE TRUE**
In diabetic ketoacidaemic coma some degree of dehydration is always present and ocular tension is lowered. Abdominal pain may be severe and nausea and vomiting are almost invariable when the ketonaemia and acidaemia are well advanced. The depth of coma is not directly related to the degree of blood glucose elevation nor does the clinical response to treatment necessarily parallel the improvement in blood glucose levels. Treatment of diabetic ketoacidaemic coma should always be centred around insulin (iv or im) and fluid replacement (iv). There is no place for sulphonylureas in the management of this acute complication. Great caution should be exercised in the use of bicarbonate infusions, and these are best avoided unless the pH is below 7.1.

27   **B**
Carriage of oxygen by haemoglobin is influenced by a number of factors. With increasing carbon dioxide tension and hydrogen ion concentration, more oxygen is released into a given tissue, i.e. the affinity is decreased. Increase in temperature has a similar effect, so that in more active tissues more oxygen is given off.
Another important factor influencing the affinity of haemaglobin for oxygen is the concentration of 2,3 diphosphoglycerate (2,3DPG), increasing concentrations leading to a reduced affinity.
The percent saturation of haemoglobin is influenced by oxygen tension, but not affinity. Serotonin has no effect.

28   **C E**
Minimal change glomerulonephritis is the most common cause of the nephrotic syndrome in children. It causes a highly selective proteinuria, and responds well to treatment (usually with high dose steroids). Patients with the nephrotic syndrome are prone to infections and thrombotic conditions.
Serum cholesterol is often raised but may be normal and is not essential for the diagnosis.

29 C D

Alphafoetoprotein is an embryonic antigen which is often secreted by hepatomas. It may be slightly raised in some forms of liver disease but substantial elevations should alert one to the diagnosis of hepatoma particularly if there is pre-existing cirrhosis.

30 A B

Patients with chronic renal failure develop a distal sensory neuropathy which may be improved by dialysis. In contrast transplantation may dramatically improve the neuropathy.

Sensorimotor neuropathy associated with isoniazid therapy may be associated with skin changes and mental symptoms and is thought to be due to pyridoxine deficiency. It appears in patients who detoxicate isoniazid slowly. Diabetic amyotropy (femoral neuropathy) is classically painful with weakness and wasting possibly due to infarction of the femoral nerve.

31 A B C D E

A third heart sound reflects rapid ventricular filling in early diastole and may be a consequence of ventricular decompensation or A-V valve regurgitation. Significant mitral stenosis prevents rapid left ventricular filling. In constrictive pericarditis the restrictive effect of the adherent pericardium halts diastolic filling abruptly, producing a third heart sound (pericardial knock).

32 A B

Farmers' lung is usually caused by *Micropolyspora faeni* which flourishes in hay which has been harvested without drying.

Breathlessness, rigors, fever and a dry cough occur two/six hours after exposure. Eosinophilia is not a feature. Diffusion capacity is reduced.

33 C D E

Phenobarbitone, phenytoin and rifampicin are potent inducers of hepatic mixed function oxidase. The clearance of the steroids is increased, the plasma concentrations fall and break-through bleeding may occur. Neither diazepam nor isoniazid induces steroid metabolism.

34 C D E

Tuberculoma of the brain may present as a dense granular calcification similar to that found in tuberculous lymph nodes.

Chest X-ray will frequently show similar calcified mediastinal nodes Calcification in the brain of a new born infant is strongly suggestive of toxoplasmosis with diffuse calcification throughout the cerebrum. Calcification in a subdural haematoma is a complication of an old head injury.

35 B D E
Cystic fibrosis is an autosomal recessive condition. Pancreatic secretions inhibit iron absorption, so that iron deficiency is very unusual in the disease, especially as patients have increased appetite.

36 D
Section 29 of the Mental Health Act (1959) allows for compulsory detention of a patient in hospital for 72 hours on the recommendation of a single Medical Practitioner and the application of an authorised Social Worker or close relative.

37 B D E
In idiopathic hirsutism the plasma testosterone level is usually mildly elevated. Phenytoin may cause a generalised increase in hair growth usually two to three months after the beginning of treatment.
Certain types of congenital adrenal hyperplasia can lead to increased androgen production, hirsutism and virilisation. Excessive production of androgens by the ovary is most commonly due to polycystic ovarian disease or ovarian hyperthecosis. There is a definite association between hyperprolactinaemia and hirsutism but the exact mechanism has not been clarified.

38 A B D E
Trichinosis is caused by *Trichinella spiralis,* normally a parasite of carnivorous animals and is usually contracted by eating undercooked meat, particularly pork or beef. After penetration of the encysted larvae into the G.I. tract migration of the larvae to the muscles causes eosinophilia, orbital oedema, muscle tenderness and subungual haemorrhages. Thrombocytopenia secondary to D I C is very rare and usually caused by gram negative septicaemia.

39 B C D
The carpal tunnel syndrome, a form of entrapment neuropathy, is most commonly seen in middle aged women who are otherwise healthy, and evidence suggests that the cross-sectional area of the carpal tunnel in these patients is relatively small. Important associations are seen with pregnancy, diabetes mellitus, acromegaly and rheumatoid arthritis.

40 B C E
Carcinoma of the oesophagus can complicate coeliac disease, Barrett's oesophagus and a caustic soda stricture of the oesophagus. It usually presents with painful progressive dysphagia.

41 B D

Pontine lesions produce contralateral hemiplegia since the pyramidal tracts have not decussated at this level. Diplopia is due to involvement of the VIth nerve and nystagmus to involvement of the pontocerebellar fibres. Hemianaesthesia would be contralateral since the sensory tracts have decussated and the tongue would be spared since the motor fibres arise from the medulla.

42 D

In a population of patients with carcinoma sputum cytology yields 70% true positive and 30% false negative results. Metastases may grow to a considerable size before ulcerating into the bronchus and giving positive results. Confusion may be caused by non-metastatic complications. Incidence is related to population smoking habits and is rising in females. Prognosis and haemoptysis are unrelated.

43 A C D E

(A) is true and may be complicated by DIC, and even in Hodgkin's is currently less popular in view of (A). Splenic atrophy may occur in all inflammatory bowel disorders. (E) is true although not affecting the presence of spherocytosis. Howell-Jolly bodies in the presence of acanthocytosis is virtually pathagnomonic of reduced splenic function.

44 A E

Aspirin inhibits platelet function; like other non-steroidal anti-inflammatory agents (including phenylbutazone but not paracetamol) it inhibits the synthesis of prostaglandins which normally protect the mucosa. Phenylbutazone decreases the clearance by metabolism of the active isomer of warfarin. By contrast phenobarbitone induces hepatic mixed function oxidase, thereby increasing warfarin clearance and reducing the response to a given dose. Diazepam does not interact.

45 A B C E

Apnoea is common in infants under three months and may occur without the cough. Suppression of paroxysms of coughing is extremely difficult in all age groups.

46 B C E

Approximately 85% of unconjugated bilirubin is derived from the breakdown of haemoglobin haem which has come from mature circulating erythrocytes. Conjugation by microsomes in the smooth endoplasmic reticulum is increased by phenobarbitone. This drug increases the activity of uridine diphosphoglucuronyl transferase which is sited mainly on the microsomes. Novobiocin jaundice is due to interference with bilirubin conjugation whereas methyltestosterone jaundice is due to interference with bilirubin excretion. In the terminal ileum and large bowel bacterial B-glucuronidases hydrolyse bilirubin before it is reduced to urobilinogen.

47 A B D
Neurological degeneration of various types occurs with ageing. Absence of abdominal reflexes and ankle jerks is normal. Vibration sense is commonly lost at the ankles. The pupil decreases in size with age but maintains its reaction to light. The presence of a grasp reflex is pathological and correlates with cortical atrophy.

48 A B C D E
Psychiatric symptomatology including depression and delusions are not uncommon in Cushing's syndrome. Physical signs include hypertension, hypertrichosis (hirsutism) and occasionally polycythaemia. The commonest cause of Cushing's syndrome before the age of 7 years is an adrenal tumour. After the age of 7 years the commonest cause in pituitary dependent disease. Short stature or poor growth velocity may be a prominent feature in childhood.

49 A B D
Onchocerciasis (river blindness) microfilaria infect the eye directly via the blood stream. *Toxocariasis* (visceral larva migrans) *nematode* larvae invade the eye. Trachoma causes visual loss by scarring of cornea and keratitis but not direct infection of the eye.
Toxoplasmosis (particularly when congenital) causes choroidoretinits. Acquired infection with the coccidian parasite, *toxoplasma gondii,* very rarely causes any problems but if visual problems occur direct infection is the mechanism. In Chaga's disease although the cornea can be the entry site for the Trypanosome, intraocular problems have not been described,

50 A C E
The course of systemic sclerosis is extremely variable. Those with life-threatening visceral involvement (renal, cardiac and pulmonary) tend to die within the first 5 years of the disease, the rest tend to survive for much longer. Oesophageal involvement and calcinosis are not unfavourable features. D-penicillamine softens affected skin but vascular disease and visceral involvement are not significantly influenced. Exposure to cold precipitates arterial vasoconstriction in the digits, lungs and kidneys and may affect the progress of the disease.

51 A B D
Chronic renal failure results from a reduced nephron population and

the diminished glomerular filtration rate causes a rise in serum creatinine. Diminished excretion of phosphate together with reduced calcium absorption from lack of secondary hydroxylation of vitamin D in the kidney, results in lowering of the serum calcium. The kidney is the primary route for acid excretion and its retention in renal failure results in acidosis and a lowering of serum bicarbonate. The acidaemia protects the patient from tetany by increasing the ionised portion of the reduced total serum calcium.

52 A

The onset of Parkinson's disease is usually between 55 and 70 and a positive family history is rare. The increase in tone is extrapyramidal, not pyramidal, and ankle clonus would suggest Parkinson's syndrome rather than disease. The tremor may be increased by chlorpromazine.

53 A B D

Recent infarction and cardiac surgery both predispose to atrial fibrillation which is usually transient. Sinus tachycardia is typical in anxiety, while in hyperthyroidism, sinus tachycardia or atrial fibrillation may occur.

54 A B C

The sciatic nerve is the largest in the body and is derived from the lumbosacral plexus (L4, 5; S1, 2 and 3). The gluteus maximus is supplied by the inferior gluteal nerve whilst the gluteus medius and minimus are supplied by the superior gluteal nerve. Although supplying the fibres inserted into the ischial tuberosity, the sciatic nerve is only secondary to the obturator innervation. The obturator nerve supplies all the adductor group of muscles including gracilis.

55 A C

When sarcoidosis presents with erythema nodosum the prognosis is very good. Hypercalcaemia is usually due to increased Vitamin D sensitivity but hyperparathyroidism should be excluded if the hypercalcaemia is present with clinically mild disease.

Corticosteroid treatment is essential for all people with ocular involvement. False positives rarely occur with the Kveim test but false negatives can occur in up to a third of patients.

56 A B C D

Treatment is immunosuppressive, and varicella/zoster produces disseminated infection, pneumonia or encephalitis. The last two are produced by measles and CMV, and the latter may produce fatal pneumonitis, hepatitis and GIT ulceration. All live vaccines are dangerous but diphtheria and tetanus toxoids may be given.

57   B E

No dose of bendrofluazide can match the maximum diuretic effect of frusemide; nor can any dose of codeine match the maximum analgesic effect of pethidine. In the other instances however the second drug can match the maximum diuretic, anti-inflammatory or analgesic effect of the first by appropriate adjustment of dose.

58   A C D

Umbilical hernia is a feature of cretinism from which Down's syndrome has to be differentiated.

59   A D E

The sample mean, median and mode will be similar but it is the population mean, median and mode that are the same in the normal distribution. Probability can never be negative. In the Binomial distribution if the probability of an event occurring is p then the probability of it not occurring is q=1-p.

60   B C D

Symptoms include weakness, fatigue, exertional dyspnoea, angina, effort syncope and sudden death. Forceful right atrial contraction is necessary to fill the hypertrophied right ventricle and the large A wave in the jugular venous pulse reflects this. Right ventricular hypertrophy is characterized by a dominant R wave in lead V1-2. Finger clubbing is not a feature.

PRACTICE EXAM 4

1   A D E

Aminophylline by slow intravenous injection is at least as effective as an agonist at β_2-adrenoceptors such as salbutamol.

Hydrocortisone can be life-saving in status asthmaticus but is slow in onset of action. Aerosol inhalation of any bronchodilator achieves poorer relief, the more severe the restriction to air flow and ipratropium is particularly slow (30-60min) in onset of action.

Penetration can be greatly assisted by IPPV.

2   A C D E

In the majority the remission may be up to 80% in those below 50 years of age, but best results still only give 1-2 year median survival. Immunotherapy using BCG and blasts may have given longer remissions but it is still an 'open' question. Survival can be prolonged

with cyclophosphamide 60mg/Kg for 2d. and 4d. 1000 Rad total body irradiation. (E) is true in allogeneic transplants.
There is an acute type which is frequently fatal and a chronic type in 30% which is fatal from 6 months onwards.

3 **B D**
The gluteus minimus muscle is supplied by the superior gluteal nerve. The femoral nerve supplies the skin over the lower medial part of the leg and medial malleolus via its saphenous branch (L4).
The femoral nerve supplies the hip and knee joints, but the ankle joint is supplied by the tibial and deep peroneal nerves.

4 **A B D**
Fine nodular calcification on chest radiographs may occur following chickenpox and histoplasmosis. Asbestosis produces diffuse fibrosis and pleural plaques. Sarcoidosis typically produces bilateral hilar lymphadenopathy.

5 **A E**
In HOCM the onset of atrial fibrillation commonly precipitates congestive cardiac failure which is poorly tolerated. The late systolic murmur is maximal at the left sternal edge. Trinitrin increases outflow obstruction. Propranolol therapy results in symptomatic improvement in many patients but it does not prevent the complication of sudden death. Echocardiography detects septal wall hypertrophy and abnormal systolic anterior motion of the anterior leaflet of the mitral valve.

6 **A C E**
Motor neurone disease is characterised by selective degeneration of motor neurones leading to muscle weakness, wasting and fasciculation. It does not give rise to sensory symptoms. The disease is twice as common in men as it is in women. Weakness of trunk, respiratory and sphincter muscles may occur in the late stages of the disease.

7 **B E**
Recognised features of hiatus hernia include acid regurgitation especially on stooping, and worsening of symptoms during pregnancy (due to mechanical factors and the smooth muscle relaxant action of progesterone). Gradual blood loss from the lower end of the oesophagus may lead to iron deficiency anaemia.

8 **A B C D**
The incidence of renal involvement in large series varies from 79 to 87% and renal failure is a common cause of death. Micro-aneurysms affecting medium sized vessels are characteristically seen during

renal and coeliac axis angiography. Eosinophilia is a pointer to hypersensititity which is thought to be aetiological in some cases and in others to be associated with hepatitis B virus. Renal biopsies show the presence of fibrin but rarely complement deposition.

9 B D E
Spontaneous bleeding into joints occurs in bleeding disorders due to deficient coagulation factors, such as in haemophilia but not in those due to thrombocytopenia. Acute post-streptococcal glomerulonephritis is not accompanied by arthritis (cf. rheumatic fever which complicates group A haemolytic streptococcal pharyngitis in about 3% of subjects). In sarcoidosis there is a characteristic syndrome of fever, polyarthralgia, erythema nodosum, bilateral hilar lymphadenopathy and sometimes acute iritis. This occurs most often in women of child-bearing age. Gonococcal bacteraemia may be associated with an immune-complex mediated polyarthritis, or a septic arthritis in one or a few joints.

10 A B
The inheritance mechanisms of both haemophilia and Duchenne muscular dystrophy are linked to the X chromosome. Inheritance of both congenital pyloric stenosis and Huntingdon's chorea is autosomal dominant. The mechanism for cystic fibrosis of the pancreas is unknown.

11 B D
Ninety per cent of all phaeochromocytomata originate in the adrenal medulla. Hypertension is a common feature and may be paroxysmal or persistent. Rarely the paroxysms are associated with hypotension. Various methods of localisation have been successful including IVP, aortography, CAT scan, but retroperitoneal insufflation is of no value. Phaeochromocytoma may be associated with medullary thyroid carcinoma and hyperparathyroidism. Preoperatively the patient is treated by a combination of α and β blockade.

12 C D
Essential tremor is common in old age and is more likely to be increased by activity and dampened by alcohol. Propranolol does reduce essential tremor. The presence of other neurological signs support Parkinsonism. In old age a positive family history is not helpful in either direction.

13 A B C
The right coronary artery is found in a groove between the right atrium and right ventricle. It gives off a branch to the A-V node and goes on to supply the inferior aspect of the left ventricle.

14   A C E

Captopril is largely inactivated by renal mechanisms. It was designed to inhibit angiotensin II production from its immediate precursor, angiotension I but has other actions. The reduced angiotensin drive to aldosterone secretion provides a potassium conserving effect. Benefit in severe heart failure accrues from reduced afterload. The hypotensive action in normotensives has prompted a re-evaluation of the physiological role of angiotensin.

15   A B C

In (A) cold antibody with anti I (red cell antigen) specificity is usual and rarely produces acute haemolysis 2 - 3 weeks after respiratory infection. Specificity in IM is anti I and may be responsible for jaundice.
(C) Chronic cold haemagglutin disease may proceed to peripheral gangrene. In (D) thermal range of antibodies is rarely above 32°C. Paroxysmal cold haemoglobinuria is a complication of syphilis.

16   B D E

The PO_2 may fall on exercise but not at rest. Lung function studies indicate a restrictive defect with reduced FVC but normal FEV1/FVC ratio, and a reduced diffusing capacity.

17   NONE TRUE

In severe aortic regurgitation from any cause the regurgitant stream may displace the anterior leaflet of the mitral valve to produce a rumbling diastolic murmur. It may be mid-diastolic and/or presystolic and is difficult to distinguishs from the murmur of mitral stenosis but in aortic regurgitation the first heart sound is not loud.

18   A B D E

Migrainous neuralgia is classically precipitated by alcohol, the attacks usually lasting two to six hours. There may be associated ptosis, ocular disturbance, corneal suffusion, increased lacrimation and nasal stuffiness on the same side and endophthalmus. The attacks are unilateral but may effect either side in different attacks.

19   B D

Human breast milk contains predominantly IgA. It provides inadequate amounts of vitamin D, the infant thus relying on hepatic stores. Infants normally consume 150 ml/Kg/day.

20   B C E

Renal failure in myeloma is characteristically associated with eosin-ophilic intratubular casts in the distal part of the nephron associated with a giant cell reaction. The glomerular abnormalities are minor even when amyloidosis occurs, as it may, in about 10% of cases. Acute renal failure may follow intravenous pyelography due to precipitation of light chains during dehydration. Hypercalcaemia may precipitate renal failure and if reversed may result in improvement in renal functioin. Uric acid crystal nephropathy can be avoided by the use of Allopurinol.

21 B

Women are affected much more commonly than men (ratio 9:1). Mouth ulceration occurs in about 20% of patients. Circulating immune complexes are not always detectable and their absence does not rule out the diagnosis. A lymphopenia is characteristic. False positive reagin tests for syphilis occur in 10 - 20% of patients with active systemic lupus erythematosus.

22 C D

30% of patients with cryptogenic tuberculosis have negative skin tests -but the diagnosis is unlikely in a 35 year old. Packed cell volume of 0.52 would be consistent with mild dehydration very common in a febrile patient. Brucellosis very rarely causes a WBC> 10,000 sometimes even neutropenia. Both myeloma and polymyalgia rheumatica are diseases of the middle age and elderly.

23 A C E

Glucagon is secreted by the pancreas in response to hypoglycaemia. It elevates blood sugar by increasing hepatic glycogenolysis (the process whereby glucogen is broken down to glucose) and hepatic gluconeogenesis (the process whereby glucose is created from non-carbohydrate molecules). The glycogenolysis is mediated by increased adenyl cyclase activity. Paradoxically insulin secretion is stimulated by glucagon. Glucagon increases the rate and force of cardiac contraction.

24 C D E

Tricyclic antidepressants are of proven value in endogenous depression but their value in reactive depression is less clear.
They are contra-indicated in acute myocardial infarctions and their side effects include weight gain and E E G changes.

25 B C D

Trigeminal neuralgia is characterised by paroxysmal brief attacks of severe pain usually in the second or third divisions of the Vth nerve. A striking feature of the attacks is that they tend to be precipitated by touching the face, talking, mastication or swallowing. Bilateral attacks are rare and the condition is slightly commoner in females than males.

26 A B C D E
If inhaled powder produces bronchospasm a bronchodilator aerosol should be used a few minutes beforehand. The mucociliary clearance of sputum is decreased by systemic administration of antagonists at muscarinic cholinoceptors and viscosity is increased. These effects are not observed with topical ipratropium. Thrush responds to topical antifungal therapy without the need to withdraw the corticosteroid. The tremor produced by agonists at β-adrenoceptors is mediated peripherally and is less distressing than the centrally mediated emetic action of methylxanthines.

27 A D E
Malignant lymphoma and C L L together provide about 5% of all paraproteins. Occasionally rheumatoid disease is associated but not scleroderma.

28 E
In acute respiratory failure the PCO_2 and hydrogen ion concentration rise. Increased bicarbonate levels indicate chronic respiratory failure. If the PCO_2 is high the PO_2 must be low unless the patient is breathing supplementary oxygen. Acidosis decreased the affinity of haemoglobin for oxygen. A low minute ventilation is the immediate cause of these changes.

29 A B C
The diastolic murmur reflects increased flow across the tricuspid valve. Splitting of the second sound is wide because of the increased volume loads on the right ventricle, and fixed because filling of the right ventricle remains constant throughout the respiratory cycle. A pulmonary ejection click is heard when there is pulmonary artery dilatation (with severe pulmonary hypertension) or pulmonary stenosis. The electrocardiogram shows RBBB with right axis deviation.

30 A B C D
Viral meningoencephalitis commonly produces seizures particularly in children whereas choriomeningitis, for example, with mumps or Coxackie rarely produces seizures except in infants. Primary hypocalcaemic or neonatal tetany is the commonest cause of hypocalcaemic fits. Tricyclic antidepressants especially Amitriptyline have epileptogenic properties and may cause fits in normal people. Trimipramine appears less epileptogenic. A flickering object with a flicker frequency of between 15 - 25 cycles per second can precipitate an epileptic fit particularly in those patients who are photosensitive on EEG. Minor

head injuries where there is no loss of consciousness do not precipitate epilepsy.

31   A C E

The disease is sero-negative by definition. The typical rash is macular. Micrognathia results from temporo-mandibular arthritis.

32   A B C D E

Biliary colic, cholecystitis and obstructive jaundice are well known complications of gall stones. 50% of stones however are silent.
Chronic haemolytic anaemias may be associated with gall stones (pigment stones) formed because of increased breakdown products of haemoglobin (pigment) excreted in the bile. Passage of a stone into the common bile duct can trigger off an attack of acute pancreatitis. An acute abdomen can be caused by acute cholecystitis or an empyema of the gall bladder due to a stone impacted in the cystic duct.

33   C D

In generalized osteoarthrosis Heberden's nodes are located at the distal interphalangeal joints and Bouchard's nodes at the proximal interphalangeal joints of the fingers. They are found most commonly in women and there may be familial aggregation. Clutton's joints are arthritic manifestations of congenital syphilis at the time of puberty. Schmorl's nodes are due to herniation of the nucleosus pulposus into adjacent vertebral bodies of the lumbar and thoracic spine. Romanus lesions are lesions at the corners of vertebral bodies in ankylosing spondylitis.

34   B E

Foxes do not carry rabies. Foxes die of rabies within 3 weeks and usually before 10 days. Sylvatic animals, moles, ground squirrels, skunks, etc. carry the disease for years. The cornea is a prominent site. 'Dumb' rabies is commoner than 'rage'. Although 'quarantine' is only 6 months incubation can be much longer in humans depending on the site of the bite.

35   C D

Phenytoin and salicylates displace thyroxine from thyroxine-binding globulin (TBG) with a resultant lowering of serum thyroxine levels. Oestrogens and clofibrate cause an increase in TBG concentration which results in a raised serum thyroxine level. Androgens lower the TBG concentration.

36   A C E

It is important to look for treatable metabolic causes of dementia such as vitamin deficiency. In Wilson's disease copper deposited in the basal ganglia and in the cortex causes Parkinsonian-like tremor and rigidity, choreoathetosis and dementia. The onset of the disease is usually in adolescence but may be delayed till adult life.

37   A C

The mode is the value that occurs most frequently. The median is the middle value, if there are an even number of values then it is the average of the 'middle two' 3.5 here. The mean is the arithmetic sum divided by the sample size. The variance is the square of the standard deviation 11-78 here. The standard error or standard error of the mean is standard deviation divided by the square root of the sample size.

38   A C E

Calcium hydroxide precipitates from the alkaline bicarbonate solution. There is no interaction between the opium alkaloids and the phenothiazines which may conveniently be injected in the same syringe. Dextrose solutions become acidic when autoclaved so that the poorly soluble phenytoin acid precipitates from the mixture.
Isophane insulin contains no excess protamine and there is no interaction with added soluble insulin. The large excess of penicillin anion forms an inactive complex with the relatively small amount of basic aminoglycoside.

39   B C E

Neurological presentation is rare except in thrombotic thrombocytopenic purpura. Fibrin deposition produces fragmentation and platelet consumption. Heparin frequently exacerbates the bleeding tendency with fatal results!

40   A B C

Lymphomas, retrosternal thyroid, terato-dermoids, pericardial cysts and aneurysms of the ascending aorta all typically occur in the anterior mediastinum. Neurogenic tumours, paravertebral abscesses and descending aneurysms are posterior.

41   C D

Splinter haemorrhages are vascular lesions due to immune complexes rather than septic microemboli. Interatrial septal defects are seldom complicated by endocarditis because they are low-pressure shunts. Left atrial myxoma may produce similar features to SABE with constitutional upset, changing murmurs and embolic manifestations.

Echocardiography is useful in excluding myxomas; also large vegetations may be detected. Microscopic haematuria is frequently present.

42   A B C E

Choreic movements may effect the mouth and jaw, trunk and respiratory muscles and in the limbs particularly the distal joints are involved. Choreic movements are increased by effort and excitement and disappear while asleep. They are often semi- purposive. Chorea may be the presenting feature of systemic lupus erythematosus and polycythaemia, and is a late presentation of phenytoin intoxication and may appear at any time in women taking the oral contraceptive pill,

43   A C E

Hypoxia occurs before hypercapnia in status asthmaticus. Careful studies have shown infants to be unresponsive to B_2 agonists.
The disease has a genetic component and significant numbers of patients wheeze throughout adolescence and become asthmatic adults.

44   A D E

Although pseudomenbranous colitis usually follows antibiotic usage there have been reports of direct person to person spread. A typical pseudomembrane is apparent on sigmoidoscopy but occasionally there is rectal sparing. As the toxin is elaborated in the gut lumen parenteral therapy is inappropriate.

45   A C D

Anaemia in C R F is largely due to lack of erythroprotein, is least marked in polycystic renal disease, and is only consistently reversed by successful renal transplantation. The degree of anaemia is broadly related to the serum creatinine, becoming manifest when the G F R falls below 30ml/min. Increased red cell 2, 3 DPG shifts the oxygen dissociation curve to the right increasing tissue oxygenation. Iron utilisation is disordered in C R F and iron deficiency is recognised by lack of stainable iron in the bone marrow or by a low serum ferritin.

46   A B D

Cyclic AMP is formed from ATP through the action of the enzyme adenylate cyclase. It mediates the action of most peptide hormones activating plasma kinase. The action is limited by phosphodiesterase which breaks down the cyclic AMP. This enzyme is inhibited by the methylxanthine caffeine and theophylline which therefore augment the action of cyclic AMP.

47   B C E

Central retinal artery occlusion from embolus or arteritis, causes sudden complete and irreversible loss of vision. Retrobulbar neuritis results in pain and temporary loss of vision. Vitreous haemorrhage, which complicates diabetic proliferative retinopathy, may be so large that effective vision is suddenly lost. Retinal detachment usually causes progressive but not necessarily rapid loss of part of the visual field. Retinitis pigmentosa is a primary retinal degeneration that produces gradual but progressive loss of vision.

48   E

Puerperal psychosis usually begins within the first 7/10 days of the puerperium and most often takes the form of depression.
Schizophrenia or mania are rare. The onset is often acute and the eventual outcome good. The risk of recurrence in subsequent pregnancies is between 1:3 and 1:7.

49   A C D

Marburg virus (Green Monkey Disease) - maculopapular rash with erythematous background is very common. ARBO viruses are athropod borne viruses. Lassa fever virus is an arena virus (looks like an arena/circle) under E M. Yellow fever and smallpox vaccine are both live vaccines but as long as they are given together, i.e. at the same time, the 'non-specific' effects of one will not interfere with the efficacy of the other. Louping ill is an arbovirus but is transmitted by ticks not mosquitoes.

50   B C E

Ankylosing spondylitis is associated with fibro-bullous disease of the apices. Pleurisy with or without effusion can complicate any collagen vascular disorder. Basal pneumonia in systemic sclerosis results from oesophageal dysfunction and aspiration. Yellow nails demonstrate a deficiency of lymphatics and the effusion is not chylous. The most frequent primaries to cause lymphangitis are stomach, pancreas, breast and prostate.

51   A B E

Hypokalaemia (occasionally occurring with prolonged use of thiazide diuretics) causes a prominent U wave, T wave flattening, and later ST depression and T wave inversion. Pericarditis causes concave upward ST elevation. The strain pattern of left ventricular hypertrophy shows ST depression and digoxin toxicity shows ST depression with the 'reversed tick' appearance.

52   C D

The primary defect in myasthenia gravis is loss of the post junctional acetycholine receptors, mediated by complement fixating antibody. Treatment is with the anticholinesterase neostigmine, but in excessive dosage, cholinergic crisis with serious respiratory paralysis can be induced. Thymectomy is undertaken for cases with and without thymoma; the prognosis for the former is worse even when the thymoma is non-malignant.

53 A C E

Hypoparathyroidism may cause the phenomenon. Craniopharyngioma is the pituitary tumour usually associated with calcification.

54 B D E

Ulcerative colitis classically involves the colon and rectum causing mucosal ulceration which, if severe enough, has a pseudopolypoid appearance. It represents islands of remaining mucosa. Diarrhoea and rectal bleeding are classical presenting symptoms. Fistula formation is more typical of Crohn's disease and cobblestoning describes the X-ray appearance of the mucosa in that disease.

55 D

Inappropriate A D H secretion is defined as excessive urinary concentration in the face of dilute plasma. Plasma/serum electrolytes and urea are all reduced and blood pressure is maintained due to water retention in contra-distinction to Addison's disease where serum potassium and blood urea are raised and blood pressure falls. It may be associated with oat cell carcinoma of the bronchus and other tumours.

56 D

Blood flow through various brain tissues varies, being relatively high in the cortex. Blood flow distribution also depends on the activity of the individual. Flow decreases with increased intracranial pressure and there is compensation for changes in arterial pressure at the level of the head, as for example, in situations of altered gravitational field. Vasomotor reflexes play little if any part in regulation of the cerebral circulation.

Flow is influenced by brain metabolism so that an increase in hydrogen ion concentration can be accompanied by an increase in blood flow.

57 A B D

Drugs such as sulphonamides or the contraceptive pill may cause erythema multiforme and virus infections especially those due to herpes simplex or *Mycoplasma pneumoniae* may be trigger factors. Erythema nodosum is associated with ulcerative colitis and erythema marginatum characterised by evanescent polycyclic erythematous rings is specific for acute rheumatic fever.

58 C D
Because of the complication of lactic acidosis, phenformin is no longer used in the treatment of diabetes mellitus. The regime for maturity onset diabetes is an oral hypoglycaemic and/or a diet. Insulin may be required for some patients who are not controlled on this regime. Glibenclamide occasionally leads to hypoglycaemic coma. In hyperosmolar coma, rehydration is the mainstay of treatment and patients tend to be sensitive to small doses of insulin. Chlorpropamide can lead to cholestatic jaundice due to hypersensitivity.

59 D E
Gastrin is produced by the argyrophil cells in the pyloric antral area and the proximal duodenum (G cells). It can also be demonstrated in normal pancreatic islet cells. Gastrin release is inhibited by antral and duodenal acidification. Gastrin acts directly on parietal cells and its effect is significantly reduced by H_2 receptor antagonists such that basal and stimulated acid output are almost completely inhibited. Serum gastrin level is elevated in pernicious anaemia where gastric acid output is absent or reduced. Gastrin is degraded in the kidney and elevated levels occur in chronic renal disease.

60 B C
The selectivity of atenolol, though significant, is less than that of practolol. There is a substantial vagal component to the reversible airways obstruction of chronic bronchitis. Elixir or soluble tablets of theophylline have an effective duration of action of 7 hours. The slow release formulation extends this to 12 hours. The non-selective agonists at β-adrenoceptors including orciprenaline are now regarded as less suitable and less safe as bronchodilators than the β_2-selective ones.
Slow intravenous infusion of corticosteroids is effective in status asthmaticus only if preceded by a bolus loading dose.

PRACTICE EXAM 5

1 A B C E
About 95% of patients with ankylosing spondylitis are HLA-B27 positive. Patients with ulcerative colitis, Reiter's syndrome and psoriasis may have sacro-iliitis and less frequently spondylitis; when

these are present the patients are usually HLA-B27 positive as well. In ulcerative colitis the sacro-iliitis and spondylitis are unrelated to the activity of the colitis and may progress following panproctocolectomy.

2   **A E**
Glycosuria is as important a diagnostic tool in old age as in younger age groups. Renal threshold tends to be high in old age.
Vulvovaginitis or balinitis in the male, which often yields candida on culture, are common and important complications of glycosuria. The significance of glycosuria needs to be confirmed by measuring blood glucose.

3   **B E**
Transient but not permanent diabetes insipidus may occur after destruction of the posterior lobe of the pituitary. Adequate circulating corticosteroids are required to excrete a water load; therefore cortisol deficiency will mask cranial diabetes insipidus which will only become apparent after steroid replacement therapy. Lithium toxicity may cause acquired nephrogenic diabetes insipidus. The treatment of choice in cranial diabetes insipidus is intranasal desmopressin. Under no circumstances should patients with untreated diabetes insipidus restrict their fluid intake as dehydration would ensue.

4   **B**
In achondroplasia because of disturbed endochondrial bone formation the base of the skull is relatively short, the sella turcica small and the foramen magnum constricted. The facial bones are normal and the cranial vault is short. There is disproportion and shortening of the long bones compared to the spine. However bone metabolism is normal with no increased incidence of spontaneous fractures. Inheritance is autosomal dominant.

5   **B C**
Herpangina is characterised by fever, sore throat and a painful vasicular enanthem on the tonsils and soft palate. It is usually caused by Group A coxsackieviruses but other enteroviruses such as coxsackie B or echoviruses may be responsible. Herpes simplex infections are caused by *Herpesvirus hominis* Type I. Apart from cold sores the commonest clinical manifestion is acute ulcerative stomatitis.

6   **B C D E**
Syringomyelia affects the lower cervical and upper thoracic spinal cord and interrupts the nerve fibres conducting pain and temperature. Proprioception is preserved. Wasting and loss of reflexes occur at the

level of the lesion (upper limbs). The lower limbs may show upper
motor neurone signs (brisk reflexes, extensor plantar response).

7   A D
Although CCU's reduce hospital mortality of AMI by about a third
most patients that die do so before reaching hospital. The risk of
pulmonary and systemic thromboembolism is significantly reduced
by anticoagulants. When complete heart block complicates anterior
myocardial infarct the mortality is high, despite a pacemaker, because
of extensive myocardial damage. Relative hypovolaemia is a not
uncommon cause of hypotension, particularly with inferior infarcts.
Diabetics have an increased risk of primary ventricular fibrillation in
the second week.

8   B C E
Precipitating antibodies against sugar cane cause type III hypersensitivity in bagassosis and similar antibodies are present in
histoplamosis and bird fancier's lung. In fibrosing alveolitis anti-IgG
and anti-nuclear factor are sometimes present. Antibodies have not
been found in byssinosis.

9   A D E
A D & E may all result in a dry tap due to increased reticulin.
Aplasia may be patchy and Reed-Sternberg cells are difficult to
identify in a hypercellular aspirate. Histology makes interpretation of
morphology of the erythroid series difficult.

10   B D
The adductor pollicis is the odd one out with regards to the small
muscles of the thumb. It is normally ulnar innervated whilst the others
are median nerve innervated, such as opponens pollicis.
The flexor pollicis longus however, will be unaffected by wrist
compression as it is innervated by the anterior interosseous nerve in
the forearm. The skin of the medial part of the ring finger will be
affected by the compression, but the thenar skin is supplied by the
palmar branch of the median nerve, which passes superficial to the
flexor retinaculum and is therefore unaffected.

11   A B C
All antipsychotic drugs are capable of causing tardive dyskinesia
though the incidence is low with thioridazine. The central actions of
metoclopramide are similar to those of the phenothiazines. In contrast
to Parkinson-like side effects, tardive dyskinesia is not directly due to
dopamine receptor blockade but is characterised by dopamine
supersensitivity.
Atropine-like drugs aggravate the condition. Another difference from

Parkinson-like side effects is that tardive dyskinesia may be irreversible. Note that the symptoms can initially be alleviated by increasing the dose of the anti-psychotic drug but this will aggravate the condition in the long term.

12   B E

Reiter's syndrome and ankylosing spondylitis belong to the seronegative spondyloarthritides. Plantar fasciitis can occur in both and calcification at the ligamentous insertions to the calcaneum may subsequently develop.

13   A C D

Approximately two-thirds of the daily production of T_3 is derived by conversion from T_4 in the periphery.

The remainder is secreted directly from the thyroid gland. T_3 toxicosis is associated with an absent TSH response to TRH. The two most important hormone estimations for the diagnosis of hypothyroidism are T_4 and TSH.

In some hypothyroid patients with a low T_4 and a raised TSH, the serum T_3 level may be normal.

The incidence of T_3 toxicosis varies in different areas of the world. However it is commoner in iodine deficient areas. The half life of T_3 is aproximately 24 hours while that of T_4 is about 7 days.

14   A B C D E

Osteoarthrosis develops secondarily when the architecture of bone is altered as in Paget's disease and in avascular necrosis of the hip (related to deep-sea diving, high-dose corticosteroid therapy and sickle-cell disease). The overgrowth of joint cartilage in acromegaly and the hypermobile, unstable joints in some types of the Ehlers-Danlos syndrome also predispose to osteoarthrosis. In Kashin-Beck disease cartilage is destroyed following the ingestion of the rye fungus, *Fusarium sporotrichiella*. It occurs in Eastern Siberia and Mongolia.

15   B D

If urine testing reveals heavy proteinuria a diagnosis of nephrotic syndrome is clear and this is occasionally seen in association with carcinoma of the bronchus. Inappropriate secretion of ADH would be expected to lower both the serum potassium and the blood urea, and the serum proteins would be reduced to much less a degree. A combination of distal tubular diuretic (i.e. Aldactone or Amiloride) and a 'proximal' diuretic (i.e. Thiazide or Frusemide) with potassium supplements is very likely to lead to this electrolyte disorder. Immediate treatment is required to remedy life threatening hyperkalaemia.

16 A C D
Koplik spots are white (grains of salt on erythematous background).
Deaths are usually due to staphylococcal pneumonia.
Giant cell pneumonia is particularly common in the immune suppressed.

17 B D
Korsakoff's psychosis typically follows an episode of delirium tremens in which thiamine deficiency is probably the major factor. However there are other causes such as head injury or brain tumour. It is usually a chronic condition though recovery is possible.
Unlike delirium there is clear consciousness and unlike more global forms of dementia intellectual capacity is relatively well preserved.

18 A B C D E
In cyanotic heart disease, especially right ventricular outflow tract obstruction, myocardial ischaemia may occur.

19 B D E
Myotonia is a continued action of muscular contraction after cessation of voluntary effort or stimulation and therefore differs from the contracture of McArdle's disease. It is not a feature of Duchenne muscular dystrophy but may be seen particularly with hyperkalaemic periodic paralysis. Procainamide and Epanutin are effective in reducing symptoms. Particularly with hereditary myotonia, the patient may have no symptoms related to the myotonia.

20 B C
Sino-atrial disease is characterized by sinus bradycardia, bradyarrhythmias and various atrial tachyarrhythmias. Ventricular dysrhythmias are uncommon. Patients with alternating tachycardia and bradycardia are at particular risk of systemic emboli and anticoagulants are advisable. Antiarrhythmic drug treatment is seldom helpful since other arrhythmias are usually induced.
Patients with troublesome symptoms should be paced, but the prognosis for those with or without pacemakers is good.

21 B C D E
Non-metastatic manifestations of carcinoma of the bronchus include cerebellar degeneration, hypercalcaemia and ectopic ACTH and MSH production.

22 A B E
In (A) there is hormonal suppression of normal cells by leukemic cells and mechanical 'crowding out' in the bone marrow. In (B) thrombocytopenia may be an initial manifestation. Septicaemia induces consumption by immune complexes, complement activation and

direct toxaemia. Massive transfusion produces thrombocytopenia by dilution.

23　A D
Metronidazole is drug of choice. Clindamycin is active against a wide variety of anaerobes including *bacteroides fragilis* and although Benzylpenicillin is effective against many anaerobes, *bacteroids fragilis* is not one of them.

24　A C E
Parkinson-like effects are brought about by dopaminergic deficit in the nigrostriatal tracts. Drugs which antagonise the action of dopamine at receptors in this area and thus produce the effects, are the neuroleptics, haloperidol, perphenazine and trifluoperazine. Imipramine is a central muscarinic antagonist of acetylcholine and phenytoin is likewise without action at dopamine receptors.

25　A B C
The common peroneal branch of the sciatic nerve winds around the neck of the fibula prior to dividing into the superficial and deep peroneal nerves. These nerves control eversion and dorsiflexion which, if lost give rise to an inverted plantar-flexed foot, i.e. foot drop. Inversion would not be completely lost as tibialis posterior is innervated by the tibial nerve and it is an invertor.
The sole of the foot is innervated by the medial and lateral plantar branches of the tibial nerve.

26　ALL FALSE
Endogenous depression usually develops gradually over a period of days or weeks. Loss of energy and marked weight loss are usual. Although psychomotor retardation is often present some patients present with the picture of 'agitated depression'. Only about 60% of cases respond to drug therapy.

27　A D
Primary hypothyroidism characterised biochemically by a raised TSH and low T_4 is a not uncommon cause of short stature. Patients with Klinefelter's syndrome are usually tall. Males with idiopathic growth hormone deficiency often have microgenitalia. In either idiopathic or acquired growth hormone deficiency gonadotrophic deficiency not infrequently co-exists. Coeliac disease in childhood may present with short stature and anaemia. A girl with Turner's syndrome (45X) will not reach a normal height unless she is a Turner's mosaic. Oestrogen therapy will not modify the eventual adult height achieved.

28   A D E
Candida albicans infection can extend from the oral cavity to the anus and oesophagitis can be severe enough to mimic varices radiologically.
Renal glycosuria unlike diabetes does not predispose to candida infection. Clotrimazole treats Candida infections very well.

29   A B C E
In the secondary forms of gout, hyperuricaemia may be due to either overproduction or underexcretion of uric acid. Myeloproliferative disorders such as PRV have an increased turnover of nucleic acids. Glycogen storage disease (type 1) is associated with increased urate production. Urate excretion is impaired in chronic renal failure although clinical gout is rare. Pseudogout due to pyrophosphate crystal arthropathy is much more common. Lead poisoning leads to gout by inhibiting the tubular secretion of uric acid. Diuretics do the same and are a much commoner precipitant of gout.

30   A B C
Oesophgeal spasm occurs in all age groups and can mimic angina closely even to the extent of being relieved by GTN. The diagnosis is suggested by a corkscrew oesophagus on barium swallow and simultaneous non-peristaltic contractions on manometry.

31   B C E
A grasp reflex is a sign of frontal lobe disorder, usually a tumour, while hemiplegia more marked in the arm than in the leg suggests a lesion of the middle cerebral artery which supplies the lateral surface of the cerebral hemisphere. Vertigo, diplopia and dysarthria are all suggestive of a brain stem lesion.

32   C
About a third of infarcts are unrecognised clinically, sometimes because the infarct is painless (especially among elderly, anaemic and diabetic patients), sometimes because the symptoms are atypical. About a third of patients operated on within three months of an infarct have a further infarct and at least half of them die, whereas the incidence of reinfarction after six months is around 5%. Vomiting occurs in about 40% of transmural infarcts and is much less common with subendocardial necrosis. The ECG changes of LBBB tend to mask electrical evidence of a myocardial infarct. The CK-MB isoenzyme is specific for heart muscle.

33   B D E
The virus is only infective in its complete form (Dane particle) which consists of the DNA core (HBc Ag) surounded by surface (HBs Ag)

antigen. The presence of e antigen correlates with infectivity. The virus can be transmitted by insects and in high endemic areas hepatoma is a very common tumour.

34 C

Pleural plaques only indicate asbestosis exposure and are not pre-malignant. Diffuse fibrosis, not pulmonary nodules are found, and bronchial carcinoma is a recognised complication of pulmonary involvement.

35 A B C D

Pancytopenia may be caused by folic acid deficiency as noted in intensive care units and pregnancy. When caused by paroxysmal nocturnal haemoglobinuria it may terminate in aplastic anaemia. In AML both crowding out and inhibition of normal haemopoiesis occur. Haemosiderosis does not produce aplasia except that occurring in terminal sideroblastic anaemia.

36 A C

Parkinsonian rigidity may be produced by poisoning with carbon monoxide and manganese and by large doses of reserpine, methyldopa and the phenothiazines (especially chlorpromazine). Mercury poisoning gives rise to a coarse tremor. The striatum derives most of its blood supply from the anterior circulation. The contraceptive pill produces chorea rather than muscle rigidity.

37 A C E

Amitriptyline and maprotiline inhibit re-uptake of noradrenaline at central synapses and hence alleviate endogenous depression. ECT probably relieves depression by causing a temporary increase in the central biosynthesis of noradremaline. Benztropine and flavoxate are both antagonists of acetylcholine at muscarinic receptors and have no effect in endogenous depression.

38 A D E

The ureter and bladder are lined with transitional epithelium whereas the vas deferens is lined with columnar epithelium. The sympathetic nerve supply to the ureter is from spinal cord segments L1 and L2. Remember that there is no sympathetic outflow below L2.

39 A B C

In approximately 25% of acromegalics the serum phosphate level is raised. The characteristic biochemical findings in hypoparathyroidism are a lowered serum calcium, raised serum phosphate and low or undetectable parathormone level. The serum phosphate level is normal in Paget's disease and low in rickets.

In chronic renal failure excretion of phosphate is impaired and the serum phosphate level is elevated.

40   A B C D E

Auto-immune thyroid disease is one of a group of organ-specific autoimmune diseases that include pernicious anaemia, Addison's disease and hypoparathyroidism. Rarer associatioins of the organ-specific autoimmune diseases include premature ovarian failure and diabetes mellitus. Vitiligo, hypopigmented rings surrounding dark naevi (halo naevi), leucotrichia, premature greying of the hair and alopecia areata are associated dermatological manifestations. Finally females with Turner's syndrome have a much higher incidence of autoimmune thyroiditis than the general population.

41   A B C D

The half and half nail is seen in renal disease and azotaemia. The proximal nail bed is white and the distal half red. Pitting, yellow discolouration, subungual thickening and onycholysis may occur in psoriasis. In subacute bacterial endocarditis splinter haemorrhages and clubbing may occur. Severe cases of alopecia areata may show pitting, ridging, thickening and occasional loss of the nails.

42   B D E

Carbon dioxide is carried in the blood as bicarbonate (65%), as carbamino compounds with haemoglobin and plasma proteins (27%) and in simple solution (8%). When the saturation of haemoglobin with oxygen increases in the lungs, hydrogen ions combine with bicarbonate to produce carbonic acid which is rapidly dehydrated to give free CO_2. In conditions of impaired diffusing capacity, oxygen diffusion is affected more than CO_2 and thus in fibrosing alveolitis, hypoxia develops rather than hypercapnia.

43   A B D E

Currently immunosuppressive regimes, in most transplant units, include corticosteroids. Complications attributed to steroid therapy include avascular necrosis of bone, most commonly the hip, cataracts producing visual impairment, and growth retardation. The latter is occasionally alleviated by alternate day therapy. Hirsutes may be related to steroids or even antihypertensive therapy (i.e. Minoxidil) but is also a common complication of Cyclosporin A, a new immunosuppressive agent which may largely replace steroids in the future. There is an increased incidence of malignancy particularly malignant lymphoma and skin cancer.

44   A B C D E

45 B C E

In peroneal muscular atrophy the clinical manifestations usually appear in the first three decades. The clinical signs occur first in the legs and may remain confined to the legs. A small percentage of patients develop wasting of the small muscles of the hands. The disease is inherited and is autosomal dominant but its expression may vary. Progression of the disease is very slow.

The patients may not be disabled even in their 70's.

46 A B C D E

HOCM is associated with labile outflow obstruction of the left ventricle. A jerky or a bisferiens carotid pulse may be palpable.

Outflow tract obstruction is worse with standing or on exercise and syncope may be precipitated in these situations. The late systolic murmur at the left sternal edge is due to outflow tract obstruction, but mitral regurgitation is usually present as well.

Ventricular hypertrophy impairs left ventricular diastolic filling and the fourth heart sound reflects increased left atrial contractility. Septal Q waves on the ECG are the consequence of massive septal hypertrophy.

47 ALL FALSE

This is a type III hypersensitivity reaction. Symptoms occur a few hours after exposure and eosinophilia is not present. The onset is over weeks or months. Rheumatoid factor may be positive in cryptogenic fibrosing aleolitis, but is not a feature of extrinsic allergic alveolitis.

48 A B D

The major pathway of paracetamol metabolism is saturated.

Glutathione helps to inactivate the toxic intermediate but cells are damaged as supplies become exhausted. Plasma paracetamol concentrations above a critical threshold 4-12 hours after ingestion indicate risks of liver cell damage. The first direct evidence of damage is a slow decay of paracetamol concentration or prolongation of the prothrombin time. Acetylcysteine at adequate concentration reactivates oxidised gluthathione but once coma is established response to any therapy is poor.

49 A B E

Busulphan produces median remissions of 2½-3 years and long term toxicity of aplasia, lung fibrosis and Addisonian syndrome.

Radiotherapy may improve symptoms from very large spleens in the late stages and hypersplenism is occasionally an indication for splenectomy.

Splenectomy, thereby removing a source of malignant clones (MRC Trial) has not been shown to improve survival or quality of life.

50   D

The vast majority (about 85%) of insomnias are secondary to psychological factors, psychiatric or physical illnesses or drug induced states. Alcohol decreases total sleep time but decreases the time required to fall asleep. Phenothiazines may cause tardive dyskinesia. Unlike narcolepsy, hypersomnia is not associated with an irresistable urge to sleep but consists of 'hangover symptoms' due to excessive sleep which may then lead the patient to feel that he needs yet more sleep.

51   A B D

Conjunctivitis causes pain, discomfort or grittiness in the eye. Subconjunctival haemorrhages are usually painless. Iritis and acute glaucoma cause both redness and pain, and ophthalmological advice is urgent. A painful white eye with no visual symptoms is likely to have a neurological basis e.g. trigeminal neuralgia, but this is very rare.

52   A D E

This indicates that the subject is capable of 6 times the exertion that would have been possible without it. Trained athletes are able to increase the oxygen consumption of their muscles to a greater degree than untrained individuals. Consequently they are capable of greater exertion without increasing lactic acid production and hence contract smaller oxygen debts for a given amount of exertion. The production of lactic acid which is inevitable with the anaerobic pathway in action results in a lowering of the pH due to an accumulation of acid. Thus the use of the anaerobic pathway is self-limiting.

53   C D E

Cystinuria is a disorder of transport of dibasic aminoacids both in the jejunum and proximal renal tubule alone, in contrast to cystinosis (Lignac-Fanconi syndrome) where widespread abnormalities of function of both proximal and distal renal tubules occur.
Cystine stones are radio-opaque due to sulphur atoms in the molecule. Penicillamine may cause heavy proteinuria. Periodic paralysis with persistent hypokalaemia may be the presenting symptom of renal tubular acidosis often confirmed by the presence of nephrocalcinosis.
Pseudo-hypo-parathyroidism is considered to be due to adenylcyclase deficiency in the renal cortex.

54   A E

Primary biliary cirrhosis and chronic active hepatitis form a spectrum of autoimmune liver disease which is more common in women. The former occurs in a slightly older age group, is characterised by a positive mitochondrial antibody and steroids are contraindicated because of major bone complications. Chronic active hepatitis usually has a positive antinuclear antibody but occasionally an antimitochondrial antibody. It responds well to steroids. DNA binding is increased in both diseases.

55   A B C E
Protection against typhoid is only recommended for visitors to areas where the disease is endemic.

56   B
The third cranial nerve supplies the levator of the eyelid, the medial, superior, inferior recti and the inferior oblique muscles.
Paralysis causes ptosis, a dilated pupil and paralysis of action of the above-named muscles. Abduction of the eye is intact because the lateral rectus responsible for this action is supplied by the 6th cranial nerve. Direct light reflex is lost as the efferent part of the reflex is via the 3rd cranial nerve.

57   A C
In sarcoidosis with erythema nodosum the Kveim test is positive in 90% of patients. Bilateral hilar adenopathy is common but pulmonary symptoms are uncommon in spite of diffuse pulmonary involvement. Cardiac problems are usually due to pre-existing disease. Bone involvement and calcium metabolism are unrelated.

58   A B D E
Diazepam and the other benzodiazepines have many of the qualitative features of the barbiturates. The difference is in their margin of safety. Tolerance and dependence to the barbiturates occur in months and to the benzodiazepines in years. The ratio between anxiolytic and respiratory depressant dose for the barbiturates is small and that for diazepam is large. When the use of diazepam is restricted to short periods the risk of barbiturate-like hazards is virtually nil. Though tolerance does develop it is not due to induction of oxidative enzymes. Thus in contrast to barbiturates diazepam does not reduce the activities of other drugs that are similarly oxidised such as the oral contraceptives and the anticoagulants.

59   D
The inter-quartile range contains 50% of the data in a sample. It is from the 25th to the 75th percentile (the median is the 50th percentile). A confidence interval is the amount of variation acceptable at a given significance level of a statistic estimated from a sample. It is usually used with means where a 95% confidence interval is the mean plus or minus two standard deviations. In a two-tailed test as in a one-

tailed test at the 5% level, statistical significance is reached if p is greater than 0.05. A scatterdiagram or scattergram can also be used to display univariate data. A guide to accurate precision is if the coefficient of variation is small i.e. less than 20%.

60   A B E
Chronic CO_2 retention leads to bicarbonate preservation by the kidney which tends to restore the arterial pH to normal. Hypokalaemia inhibits the production of an alkaline urine in the presence of a systemic alkalosis and this may be of particular clinical significance in the treatment of aspirin poisoning. When urine is presented to the sigmoid colon chloride is preferentially reabsorbed resulting in a relative lowering of plasma bicarbonate.
Conversely excessive chloride depletion which may occur during vomiting from pyloric stenosis may cause profound alkalosis and reduction in the ionized component of calcium. Congenital adrenal hyperplasia associated with 21 Hydroxylase deficiency is usually associated with diminished cortisol production and the plasma bicarbonate is normal or reduced.

RECOMMENDED READING AND REFERENCE LIST

The following reading list has been compiled as representing the most commonly used and most valued texts by a group of physicians in training.

Many have used one of the shorter general medical textbooks as a basis for study and supplememnted this with a well established text from each of the different medical specialities. This has been of greater benefit than attempting to absorb the contents of a large reference textbook, the different sections of which are not always of the same standard.

Some have found that writing their own set of short revision notes, abstracting the information from 2 or 3 textbooks of slightly different style, has been of considerable value, the art of condensing and writing itself acting as an aid to the memory.

SHORTER TEXTBOOKS

Rubenstein D. & Wayne D. **Lecture Notes on Clinical Medicine** 2nd ed. 1982 Blackwell.

Houston J.C., Joiner C.L., Trounce J.R. **A Short Textbook of Medicine** 7th ed. 1982 Hodder and Stoughton.

MacLeod J. **Davidson's Principles and Practice of Medicine** 14th ed. 1984 Churchill Livingstone.

SHORT TEXTBOOKS ON SPECIALISED TOPICS

Concise Medical Textbooks Series Bailliere Tindall

Cardiology	D.G. Julian
Dermatology	Pegum J.S. & Harvey Baker
Gastroenterology	I.A.D. Bouchier
Psychiatry	W.H. Trethowan
Renal Medicine	Roger Gabriel
Respiratory Medicine	David C. Flenley

Lecture Notes Series Blackwell Scientific Publications

Cardiology	Fleming & Braimbridge
Dermatology	Solomon
Endocrinology	Fletcher
Geriatrics	Coni, Davison & Webster
Infectious Diseases	Warin, Ironside & Mandal
Psychiatry	Willis
Neurology	Draper
Medical Statistics	Petrie
Respiratory Disease	Brewis
Ophthalmology	Trevor-Roper

Burton J.L. **Aids to Postgraduate Medicine** 4th ed. 1983   Churchill Livingstone.
Mason & Currey. **Clinical Rheumatology** 3rd ed. 1980 Pitman.
Matthews W.B. and Miller Henry. **Diseases of the Nervous System** 4th ed. 1982 Blackwell.
Sneddon I.B. Church R.E. **Practical Dermatology** 4th ed. 1983 Arnold.
Swinscon T.D.V. **Statistics at Square One** BMJ publications.
Thompson R.B. **A Short Textbook of Haematology** 6th ed. 1984 Churchill Livingstone.

REFERENCE TEXTBOOKS

General (use one of these).
Cecil's **Textbook of Medicine** Beeson, McDermott, Wyngaarden 18th ed. 1988 Saunders.
Harrison. **Principles of Internal Medicine** 11th ed. 1986 McGraw Hill.
Textbook of Medicine, 2nd ed. 1987 Oxford University Press.

Basic Science
Ganong. **Medical Physiology** 14th ed. 1989. Lange.
Gray's Anatomy 37th ed. 1989 Longmans.

Clinical Chemistry
Zilva J.F. & Pannall. **Clinical Chemistry in Diagnosis and Treatment** 5th ed. 1988 Lloyd Luke.

Endocrinology
L. J. De Groot. **Endocrinology.** 2nd ed. 1988 Saunders.
Hall, Anderson, Smart & Besser. **Fundamentals of Clinical Endocrinology** 3rd ed. 1981 Pitman.

Gastroenterology
Sherlock S. **Diseases of the Liver and Biliary System** 7th ed. 1985 Blackwell Scientific.
Sleisenger & Fordtran. **Gastrointestional Disease** 4th ed. 1988 Saunders.
Truelove & Reyrell. **Diseases of the Digestive System** 3rd ed. 1984 Blackwell Scientific.

Haematology
De Gruchy G. **Clinical Haematology in Medical Practice** 5th ed. 1989. Blackwell Scientific.

Infectious Diseases
Christie A.B. **Infectious Diseases** 4th ed. 1987 Churchill Livingstone.

Nephrology
Black D.A.K. **Renal Disease** 4th ed. 1979 Blackwell.

Neurology

Brain. **Diseases of the Nervous System** 9th ed. 1985. Oxford University Press.

Brain. **Clinical Neurology** 6th ed. 1985 Oxford University Press.

Paediatrics

Forfar & Arneil. **Textbook of Paediatrics** 3rd ed. 1984 Churchill Livingstone.

Nelson W.E. **Textbook of Paediatrics** 13th ed. 1987 Saunders.

Psychiatry

Gelder, Gath, Majou. **Oxford Textbook of Psychiatry** 2nd ed. 1989 Oxford University Press.

Respiratory

Crofton J. Douglas A. **Respiratory Diseases** 4th ed. 1989 Blackwell.

Pharmacology and Therapeutics

Goodman & Gilman. **The Pharmacological Basis of Therapeutics** 7th ed. 1985 Macmillan.

Laurence D.R., Bennett P.N. **Clinical Pharmacology** 6th ed. 1987 Churchill Livingstone.

Martindale. **Extra Pharmacopoeia** 29th ed. 1989. Pharmaceutical Press.

Rheumatology

Copeman W.S.C. **Textbook of Rheumatic Diseases** (2 vols) 6th ed. 1986. Churchill Livingstone.

Kelley, Harris, Ruddy, Sledge. **Textbook of Rheumatology** 2nd ed. 1985 Saunders.

Statistics

Bradford Hill. **A Short Textbook of Medical Statistics** 1985 Hodder & Stoughton.

JOURNALS

Medicine International Series I. II and III
British Journal of Hospital Medicine
Hospital Update
British Medical Journal ⎫
Lancet ⎭ **Leading articles**

MCQs LISTED BY SUBJECT

For those candidates who like to revise subject by subject using our suggested reading and reference list, the following lists of MCQs classified by subject may be of assistance in covering a specific subject area. (Many MCQs combine 2 subject areas but have only been listed under one category). The first number denotes which practice exam is referred to, the following number is the question number.

Eg. 3.43 = Practice Exam 3 question number 43.

NEURO.	PHARM.	RESP.	CARDIOL.	ENDO.	HAEM.	PAEDS.
1.8	1.17	1.7	1.32	1.2	1.23	1.1
1.15	1.24	1.16	1.39	1.12	1.28	1.44
1.22	1.35	1.33	1.51	1.18	1.34	1.57
1.31	1.38	1.52	1.58	1.26	1.53	2.10
1.50	1.54	1.59	1.60	2.6	2.13	2.24
1.55	2.1	2.2	2.4	2.16	2.28	2.38
2.3	2.14	2.20	2.12	2.31	2.42	2.55
2.11	2.29	2.27	2.26	2.48	2.50	3.11
2.25	2.43	2.41	2.40	3.2	2.58	3.35
2.39	2.59	2.57	2.56	3.26	3.9	3.45
2.44	3.10	3.8	3.7	3.37	3.21	3.58
2.60	3.22	3.20	3.19	3.48	3.43	
3.6	3.33	3.32	3.31	4.11	3.56	
3.18	3.44	3.42	3.53	4.23	4.2	
3.30	3.57	3.55	3.60	4.35	4.15	
3.34	4.1	4.4	4.5	4.58	4.27	
3.4	4.14	4.16	4.17	5.3	4.39	
3.52	4.26	4.28	4.29	5.13	5.9	
3.54	4.38	4.40	4.41	5.27	5.22	
4.3	4.60	4.50	4.51	5.40	5.35	
4.6	5.11	5.8	5.7		5.49	
4.18	5.24	5.21	5.20			
4.25	5.37	5.34	5.32			
4.30	5.48	5.47	5.46			
4.42	5.58	5.57				
4.52						
5.6						
5.10						
5.19						
5.31						
5.36						
5.45						
5.56						

RENAL.	GASTRO.	RHEUM.	PSYCH.	PHYSIOL.	INF.DIS.	ANAT.	DERM.
1.3	1.19	1.4	1.10	1.29	1.20	1.6	1.40
1.21	1.27	1.13	1.14	1.45	1.42	1.9	2.33
1.30	1.37	1.46	1.56	1.48	2.34	2.32	3.1
1.47	1.49	2.21	2.15	2.7	2.51	3.12	4.57
2.8	2.9	2.35	2.30	2.19	3.38	4.13	5.41
2.22	2.23	2.52	2.49	3.15	3.49	5.25	
2.36	2.37	3.14	3.13	3.27	4.22	5.38	
2.53	2.54	3.23	3.25	4.46	4.34		
3.4	3.5	3.39	3.36	4.56	5.16		
3.16	3.17	3.50	4.24	5.42	5.23		
3.28	3.29	4.9	4.36	5.52	5.28		
3.51	3.40	4.21	4.48				
4.8	4.7	4.33	5.17				
4.20	4.32	5.1	5.26				
4.45	4.44	5.12	5.50				
4.55	4.54	5.14					
5.15	5.30	5.29					
5.43	5.33						
5.53	5.54						
5.60							

STATISTICS	GENETICS	METAB.	GERIATRICS	TROP.MED.	OPHTH.
1.36	1.41	1.5	1.11	1.43	1.25
2.45	2.18	2.5	2.47	2.46	2.17
3.59	3.3	3.46	3.47	3.24	4.47
4.37	4.10	4.59	4.12	4.49	5.51
5.59	5.4	5.39	5.2		

REVISION INDEX

Each item in this index refers to a specific reference contained in a question in this book. The exam number is given first, followed by the question number ie 3.7 refers to practice exam 3 question 7.

A

acetylcholine 2.19
achondroplasia 5.4
acidosis
respiratory 4.28
acromegaly 1.18, 2.16, 5.14, 5.39
alcoholism 3.18
alopecia
areata 2.33
alphafoetoprotein 3.29
amyloidosis 2.2, 2.9, 2.58, 3.39
anaemia
aplastic 5.9
autoimmune haemolytic 1.34
iron-deficiency 2.28
pernicious 1.23, 2.13, 2.37
sideroblastic 1.53
angioid streaks 1.4
ankylosing spondylitis 5.1, 5.12
anorexia nervosa 1.10
aorta
arch 1.6
aortic regurgitation 2.12
artery
right coronary 4.13
vertebral 2.32
arthritis - see separate conditions
asbestosis 5.34
ascites 2.54
asthma 4.1, 4.26, 4.23
atrial
fibrillation 3.53
septal defect 4.29
Austin Flint murmur 4.17

B

bacteroides fragilis 5.23
benign intracranial hypertension 1.25
bicarbonate plasma 5.60
bilirubin 3.46
blindness 4.47
brain 4.56
bronchiectasis 1.62
bronchiolitis 3.11
bronchus - see lung
brucellosis 4.22, 5.35

C

calcium 1.47
urinary 1.47
campylobacter jejuni 3.17
candida 5.28
carbon dioxide 5.42
carcinoid syndrome 1.19
carcinoma - see under various organs
cardiomyopathy
alcoholic congestive (COCM) 1.58
hypertrophic obstructive (HOCM) 4.5, 5.46
carpal tunnel syndrome 3.39, 5.10
cerebrovascular disease 2.25
Chagas' disease 3.49
Charcot-Marie tooth disease 5.45
chest pain 4.18
chest X-ray 1.52, 4.4
Cheyne-Stokes breathing 2.27
child battering 1.14
chlamydia 2.53
chondrocalcinosis 1.46
chorea 4.42
chlamidia 1.30
circulation 4.56
clinical trials 1.36
clinical trials - see also statistics
coeliac disease 1.37, 2.10
cold agglutinins 4.15
complement 2.50
Crohn's disease 1.27, 2.23
CSF 2.39
Cushing's syndrome 3.48
cyclic AMP 4.46
cystic fibrosis 3.35

D

delirium tremens 2.15, 3.18
dementia 3.25, 4.36
depression 2.30, 5.26, 5.37
dermatitis herpetiformis 3.1
exfoliative 3.1
diabetes insipidus 2.31, 5.3
diabetes mellitus 1.49, 4.58
ketoacidosis 3.26
diarrhoea 2.1

disseminated intravascular coagulation 4.39
diverticular disease 3.5
Down's syndrome 3.58
drugs - see also poisoning
drugs
  acetylator status 3.10
  androgens 4.35
  antibiotics
    see also under separate names
  antidepressants
    tricyclic 4.24
  aspirin 3.21, 3.44, 3.57
  bendrofluazide 3.57
  benzodiazepines 1.54, 5.58
  beta-blockers 2.14, 4.60
  bromocriptine 2.6
  bumetanide 3.57
  captopril 4.14
  chloroquine 2.17
  clindamycin 5.23
  clofibrate 4.35
  codeine 1.38, 3.57
  contraceptives 3.33
  digoxin 2.40, 3.22
  doxycycline 2.1
  frusemide 3.57
  glyceryl trinitrate 3.19
  haloperidol 5.24
  hyoscine 1.24
  indomethacin 3.57
  insulin - see separate entry
  ipratropium 4.60
  isoniazid 3.30
  methadone 3.57
  metronidazole 5.23
  minoxidil 2.29
  morphine 3.57
  oestrogens 4.35
  oxyphenbutazone 3.21
  pentazocine 1.38
  perphenazine 5.24
  pethidine 3.57
  phenobarbitone 3.33, 3.44
  phenylbutazone 3.44
  phenytoin 3.33, 4.35 ~
  prednisolone 2.43
  procainamide 5.19
  rifampicin 1.29, 3.33
  salbutamol 4.60
  salicylates 4.35
  sulphasalazine 2.59
  theophylline 4.60
  trifluoperazine 5.24
  vasopressin - see separate entry
  warfarin 3.44

E

ebola virus disease 4.49
ECG
  ST depression 4.51
Ehlers-Danlos syndrome 5.14
encephalitis 1.42
endocarditis 3.7, 4.41
epilepsy 4.30
  temporal lobe 1.50
erythema multiforme 3.1, 4.57
erythema nodosum 2.9
extrinsic allergic alveolitis 5.47

F

Fallot's tetralogy 1.38
farmer's lung 3.32
ferritin 2.28
fibrosing alveolitis 2.20

G

galactorrhoea 1.18
gall stones 4.32
gastrin 2.37, 4.59
glomerulonephritis 3.51
  membraneous 2.36
glucagon 5.23
gonorrhoea 4.9
Goodpasture's syndrome 3.21
gout 5.29
  pseudo-gout 1.46
Grave's disease 1.2
gynaecomastia 2.18, 2.40

H

haemoglobin 3.27
haemophilia 4.9, 4.10
haemosiderinuria 1.34
headache 2.3
heart - see also myocardial infarction
heart
  failure 1.32
  left ventricular failure 1.32
  physiology 2.7
heart sound
  third 3.51
hepatitis
  B virus 5.33
herpangina 5.5
herpes simplex 5.5
hiatus hernia 4.7
hirsutism 3.37
Hodgkin's disease 5.9
Horner's syndrome 1.16

hyper-betalipoproteinaemia 1.29
hyper-cholesterolaemia 1.29
hypercalcaemia 1.4, 4.20
hyperkalaemia 1.18
hyperprolactinaemia 2.16
hyperuricaemia 2.5
hypochondriasis 1.56
hypoparathyroidism 2.48, 5.39
hypothermia 2.47
hypothyroidism 1.12
hysteria 3.13

I

infant feeding 4.19
infectious mononucleosis 4.15
inheritance
   autosomal dominant 3.3
   x-chromosome 4.10
insulin 1.26
intracranial calcification 3.54, 4.53

J

jaundice 1.17
jugular venous pulse
   cannon waves 2.4
juvenile arthritis 4.31

K

kidneys - see also under renal
kidneys
   enlarged 3.16
Klinefelter's syndrome 2.18
Korsakoff's psychosis 2.15, 5.17

L

lassa fever 4.49
Legionnaires' disease 2.51, 3.20
leptospirosis 1.20
Lesch-Nyhan syndrome 2.5
leukaemia
   acute lymphoblastic 3.57
   acute myeloid 4.2
   chronic granulocytic 5.49
   chronic lymphocytic 1.28, 4.27
   chronic myelocytic 1.28
light reflex 1.31
liver
   disease 1.5, 5.54
lung - see also under pulmonary & respiratory
lung
   abscess 1.33
   carcinoma 3.42, 5.21
   diffuse interstitial fibrosis 4.16

immunology 5.8
   physiology 1.48
lymphangitis-carcinomatosa 4.50
lymphogranuloma venereum 2.53
lymphoma 4.27
   non-Hodgkin 2.42

M

malabsorption 2.55
malaria
   falciparum 2.46
Marburg virus disease 4.49
measles 5.16
mediastinum
   anterior 4.40
Meig's syndrome 2.54
meningitis
   bacterial 2.38, 2.39
   tuberculous 2.39
Mental Health Act section 29 3.36
migrainous neuralgia 4.18
mitral
   regurgitation 2.26
motor neurone disease 4.6
mumps 2.34
muscular dystrophy
   Duchenne 1.8, 4.10
myasthenia gravis 1.15, 4.52
mycoplasma pneumoniae 4.15
myelofibrosis 5.9
myeloma 2.58, 4.20
myocardial infarction 5.7, 5.32
myotonia 5.19
myxoedema 1.23, 3.39

N

nephritis
   acute 1.3
nephrotic syndrome 3.28
nerve
   3rd cranial 5.56
   common peroneal 5.25
   femoral 4.3
   median 2.60
   radial 1.22, 2.60
   sciatic 3.54
   ulnar 2.60
neuralgia
   trigeminal 4.25
neurofibromatosis 2.44

O

oesophagus
   carcinoma 3.40

spasm 5.30
onchocerciasis 3.49
osteoarthrosis 4.33
osteomalacia 1.5, 1.11, 1.49
osteopetrosis 1.11
osteoporosis 1.11
  circumscripta 1.4
overdose - see poisoning
oxygen debt 5.52

P

Paget's disease 1.4, 1.11, 5.15, 5.39
Pancoast tumour 1.16
pancreatitis
  chronic 1.49
pancytopenia 5.35
papilloedema 1.25
paraproteinaemia 4.27
Parkinson's disease 3.52, 5.36
paroxysmal nocturnal haemoglobinuria 5.35
pericarditis 1.51
phaeochromocytoma 4.11
pneumoconiosis 2.41
pneumocystis carinii 3.8
poisoning
  drugs 1.35, 4.48
polyarteritis nodosa 4.8
polycythaemia 3.9
polymyalgia rheumatica 1.55, 2.35
polyneuropathy 3.30
pseudomembraneous colitis 4.44
psoriasis 5.1
puerperal psychosis 4.28
pulmonary - see also lung
pulmonary
  disease 4.50
  hypertension 3.60

R

rabies 4.34
Raynaud's phenomenon 4.15
rectal bleeding 5.44
regional enteritis - see also Crohn's disease
Reiter's syndrome 1.13, 5.1, 5.12
renal artery stenosis 2.22
renal - see also kidney
renal failure 4.20, 5.39
renal
  anaemia 4.45
  chronic 3.51
renal papillary necrosis 3.4
renal transplantation 5.43
renal tubular disorders 5.53

respiratory distress syndrome
  prematurity 1.57
respiratory failure 2.57
rheumatic fever 1.60
rheumatoid arthritis 2.52, 3.14, 3.23, 3.39
rheumatoid factor 2.21
rickets 5.39

S

sarcoidosis 1.47, 3.55, 4.9, 5.47
schistosomiasis 3.24
scurvy 3.21
short stature 5.17
sick sinus syndrome 5.20
spherocytosis
  congenital 1.53
splenoctomy 3.43
statistics
  binomial distribution 3.59
  chi-squared test 2.45
  confidence interval 5.59
  inter quartile range 5.59
  Mann-Whitney U-test 2.45
  mean 3.59, 4.37
  median 3.59, 4.37
  mode 3.59, 4.37
  Pearson correlation 2.45, 4.23
  scatter diagram 5.59
  standard error of the mean 4.37, 4.48
  student's unpaired test 2.45
  variance 3.59, 4.37
Stevens-Johnson syndrome 3.1
suicide 2.49
syphilis 1.21
syringomyelia 5.6
systemic lupus erythematosus 4.21
systemic sclerosis 3.50, 4.57

T

tardive dyskinesia 5.11
thalassaemia 2.24
thrombocytopenia 3.21, 5.22
thrombosis
  posterior inferior cerebellar artery 1.9
thyroid
  autoimmune disease 5.40
  carcinoma 3.2
  gland 1.3
thyrotoxicosis 2.16
toxoplasmosis 3.49
trachoma 3.49
tremor 4.12
tri iodothyronine 5.13
tropical sprue 1.23

tuberculosis 4.22
  chemotherapy 1.7
  pulmonary 1.1
Turner's syndrome 1.41
typhoid fever 1.43

U

ulcerative colitis 1.27, 2.9, 4.54, 5.1
ureter 5.38
urinary
  infection 2.8
urobilinogen 1.45

V

vaccination 5.55
Von Willebrand's disease 3.21

W

warts
  seborrihoeic 1.40
whooping cough 3.45
Wilson's disease 1.5, 4.36

Y

yellow fever 4.49

Z

Zollinger-Ellison syndrome 2.37

Royal Colleges of Physicians

SURNAME

INITIALS

Please use 2B PENCIL only. Rub out all errors thoroughly.
Mark rectangles like ▬ **NOT** like this ∕ ⊄ ✗

T ▭ = **TRUE**   F ▭ = **FALSE**   DK ▭ = **DON'T KNOW**

EXAMINATION NO.

[0]	[0]	[0]	[0]
[1]	[1]	[1]	[1]
[2]	[2]	[2]	[2]
[3]	[3]	[3]	[3]
[4]	[4]	[4]	[4]
[5]	[5]	[5]	[5]
[6]	[6]	[6]	[6]
[7]	[7]	[7]	[7]
[8]	[8]	[8]	[8]
[9]	[9]	[9]	[9]

	A	B	C	D	E			A	B	C	D	E
1	T F DK	T F DK	T F DK	T F DK	T F DK		**16**	T F DK	T F DK	T F DK	T F DK	T F DK
2	T F DK	T F DK	T F DK	T F DK	T F DK		**17**	T F DK	T F DK	T F DK	T F DK	T F DK
3	T F DK	T F DK	T F DK	T F DK	T F DK		**18**	T F DK	T F DK	T F DK	T F DK	T F DK
4	T F DK	T F DK	T F DK	T F DK	T F DK		**19**	T F DK	T F DK	T F DK	T F DK	T F DK
5	T F DK	T F DK	T F DK	T F DK	T F DK		**20**	T F DK	T F DK	T F DK	T F DK	T F DK
6	T F DK	T F DK	T F DK	T F DK	T F DK		**21**	T F DK	T F DK	T F DK	T F DK	T F DK
7	T F DK	T F DK	T F DK	T F DK	T F DK		**22**	T F DK	T F DK	T F DK	T F DK	T F DK
8	T F DK	T F DK	T F DK	T F DK	T F DK		**23**	T F DK	T F DK	T F DK	T F DK	T F DK
9	T F DK	T F DK	T F DK	T F DK	T F DK		**24**	T F DK	T F DK	T F DK	T F DK	T F DK
10	T F DK	T F DK	T F DK	T F DK	T F DK		**25**	T F DK	T F DK	T F DK	T F DK	T F DK
11	T F DK	T F DK	T F DK	T F DK	T F DK		**26**	T F DK	T F DK	T F DK	T F DK	T F DK
12	T F DK	T F DK	T F DK	T F DK	T F DK		**27**	T F DK	T F DK	T F DK	T F DK	T F DK
13	T F DK	T F DK	T F DK	T F DK	T F DK		**28**	T F DK	T F DK	T F DK	T F DK	T F DK
14	T F DK	T F DK	T F DK	T F DK	T F DK		**29**	T F DK	T F DK	T F DK	T F DK	T F DK
15	T F DK	T F DK	T F DK	T F DK	T F DK		**30**	T F DK	T F DK	T F DK	T F DK	T F DK

PRINTING AND PROCESSING BY DRS DATA & RESEARCH SERVICES PLC/I17100988

Reproduced with the kind permission of the Royal College of Physicians.

Notes

Notes